Healthy Body,
Healthy Weight,
Healthy Mind:
In Five Easy Steps

Susie Bailey

Healthy Body Healthy Weight Healthy Mind: In Five Easy Steps.
Copyright © 2016, Susie Bailey BSc (Hons)

Cover designed by Diane Hope of Print Revolution and Susie Bailey.

ISBN: 978-1-326-66770-2

PublishNation
www.publishnation.co.uk

For mum, my sons and daughters-in-love,
Mary, and all those with chronic disorders.
With love x

Acknowledgements

I would like to thank my wonderful loving family and friends, for all their support and encouragement.

Thanks also to Elaine for helping me to decide the final book title, John Armour, Professor of Human Genetics, for reviewing my research references, mum for proofreading, Diane of Print Revolution for the book cover, and Gwen of PublishNation for her skill, guidance and patience in preparing this book for publication and distribution.

Contents

Foreword

Cutting edge research over the last decade reveals the root cause of your long term health problems. This book gives you the revolutionary way to achieve a healthy body, healthy weight and a healthy mind, free of chronic disease.

If you are suffering from a chronic disorder, or want to ensure that you don't get one, this book is for you.

Chronic disorders (disorders that last longer than three months), ranging from **obesity, Alzheimer's disease, asthma** and **allergies, rheumatoid arthritis** and **Irritable bowel problems**, to **multiple sclerosis, thyroid problems, diabetes**, and **cardiovascular disease** are on the rise, but that needn't be the case. A few simple changes can transform your life; preventing, and reversing, many chronic disorders, leading to a healthy body, healthy weight, healthy mind and also a healthy wellbeing.

I use the word 'disorder', rather than disease, because, in most cases, chronic disorders don't just appear in your life, like infections, but are built up over a period of time; with symptoms gradually becoming worse until they reach a high enough level to be given the name of a specific 'disease,' like type 2 diabetes. In reality, research shows that the levels of these symptoms can also be reduced and even reversed in many cases, and so rather than having a disease, you have a temporary malfunction, which can be reversed. In other words, you can get back 'order' out of the 'disorder'. This book explains how.

I have used my honours degree in human medical genetics, and my research skills in both science and law, to research the science behind this increasing health problem; and I am passing on my findings to you, in an unbiased manner, without any agenda. This is evidence based, not just opinion. I read three thousand peer-reviewed research papers in order to write this this book, and include a few hundred of them in the references at the back of this book, together with a few articles of interest.

Many of our long term health problems are associated with the trillions of bacteria that live in our gut; but, although that is a large part of the jigsaw puzzle of long term health, other factors also contribute.

My eighteen months of research, reading thousands of published papers meant that I was able look at the overall picture; how all of the factors that have been researched contribute to long term health problems. I joined the random dots and the whole picture was revealed. More importantly, my research also showed me that there are solutions. You can reverse and prevent long term health problems, and this book takes you through the steps you need to do that. So before I continue, I'd like to say don't despair! This book has been written to empower you; to give you the tools to achieve a healthy body, healthy weight, healthy mind and healthy wellbeing.

Introduction

I first came across the possibility of reversing and preventing chronic disorders when I discovered the pioneering work of Dr A Fasano. While most doctors are taught that autoimmune and many chronic disorders are due to a person's genes, maintaining that once started the process cannot be reversed; Dr Fasano found that if we find and remove the triggers (the root causes) of an autoimmune disorder (like removing gluten for people with coeliac disease for example), it will go into remission, in spite of having those genes. (Remission means that the person is essentially cured, but if they re-introduce the trigger for that disorder it will return. In other words, if a person who has healed themselves of coeliac disease re-introduces gluten into their diet, their coeliac disease will return).

In some disorders, just *one* simple thing can act as a trigger (for example, eating gluten can cause (trigger) coeliac disease in some people), but, although books have been written for *specific* disorders (like underactive thyroid for example) I found that, although they all share the same root causes, there has not been a book written yet which explains how to find and remove the triggers of *all* chronic disorders, so I wrote this book.

I aim to show that there are five basic steps you can take to prevent and even reverse chronic disorders, as you remove the root causes of *all* long term health problems; and how you can easily fix them. I explain why, when we focus on symptoms, and the part of our body that is affected, our focus is too narrow; seeing only one small dot of information. As I just mentioned, but it is worth repeating, taking these steps will also prevent any other chronic disorders from occurring, as they share root causes. This is important because if you have one chronic disorder the chances of getting another are high (for example, people with coeliac disease may also develop an

1

underactive thyroid). Remove the root causes and you reduce that risk.

I will pass on the revolutionary understanding of our physical and mental health, joining the dots to form the whole picture. Our whole body is dynamic; constantly giving and receiving messages, and I will explain how the key systems in our body interact with each other; and how, by making a few simple easy changes, you can prevent and reverse chronic disorders.

There are **five key systems** *in* your body that are major players in your long term health; and these are

- Your DNA
- Digestion
- Your immune system
- Your gut bacteria and
- Your brain

All of these interact with each other dynamically; adjusting their responses in order to keep us healthy (or try to!). Although we have many other systems in our body, which all interact with the above and with each other, the reason why these are the *key* systems is that they are the main players when determining the bigger picture of our long term health. For example, many of the triggers for chronic disorders come from some foods, and so our digestive system is a key player as it comes into direct contact with the food.

The final piece of the jigsaw, later in the book, will explain how this dynamic interaction also includes *external* factors; including our diet, our environment, our lifestyle, and even our state of mindfulness; in a way that has never been known until now. This can be found in the chapter on solutions; and so I will call this **your sixth 'key system'**. I explain how the five key systems contribute to your health throughout the book, but mainly in the chapter on solutions, where you can also find your five step plan.

The broader picture is difficult to write about, but please bear with me, as this book gives you the information to prevent and reverse most common long term disorders; which traditional medicine, and medication, cannot cure.

Two long term disorders that have been proven to be reversible already are type 2 diabetes and coeliac disease. I will show how all chronic disorders, no matter what name we give them, all have the same root causes; and how we can fix them in five easy steps.

What I aim to do in this book is to join the dots of some amazing research, giving you the very simple information which will empower you, and enable you to transform your life; especially if you have any of the following, or want to prevent them:

Digestive problems, bloating, diarrhoea, constipation, irritable bowel syndrome, seasonal allergies, food allergies or intolerances, asthma, eczema, psoriasis, acne, hormone imbalances, pre-menstrual tension, rheumatoid arthritis, multiple sclerosis, thyroid disorder, coeliac disease, diabetes, obesity, food cravings, chronic fatigue, depression, anxiety, sleep problems, attention deficit disorder, epilepsy or have a family history of Alzheimer's disease.

Over the last ten years there has been a rapid rise in the amount of credible scientific research for chronic disorders, like the ones mentioned above, but most of the amazing findings haven't filtered into medicine yet, as it takes on average 15 years from a peer-reviewed scientific paper being published, to the findings being put into medical practice. This is not necessarily a bad thing, but conventional medicine tends to rely mainly on the research into new *pharmaceutical drugs*, funded by pharmaceutical companies, rather than any other potential solutions raised by research, and this is a costly and time consuming process. In fact, the cost of research is often a limiting factor into finding alternative solutions to pharmaceutical drugs; however, much of the research in this book suggests remedies that you can do yourself. It may also surprise you to know that pharmaceutical drugs only have to be 15% effective to be passed as offering 'treatment' (in other words they improve rather than cure a disease) whereas research shows that simple easy measures, taken by individuals, can completely **prevent** and even **reverse** chronic disorder *without* drugs, and the benefits are vast.

I will point out here that I am not anti-pharmaceuticals *per se*, as they do an amazing job for acute disorders, but some may not be helpful for either treating or preventing most *chronic* disorders; which are caused, in the main, by environmental factors which can be changed or removed. However, the first step is always to be diagnosed by a doctor and then to get any medications needed at an optimal level. After that, taking measures to heal yourself can be done, checking diagnostic markers and symptoms with your doctor as you progress together. We cannot heal all chronic disorders with western medication, but we may not always heal naturally without some help from medications, and so often need a combination of both; at least while we heal.

As I, my sons, and my mother, suffered from some of these chronic disorders I began my research to help us all, where conventional medicine could not. I found that the most surprising area of research, which is providing answers, lies in our gut. To be precise, the complex relationship we have with our gut microbes! Even more amazing is that it isn't just gut health that is affected. New emerging research is now linking our gut microbes with many chronic disorders in the body, and even to disorders associated with the brain, like Alzheimer's disease. Many disorders that the medical profession thought were untreatable are now being treated, and many disorders are being prevented and reversed.

Time to start joining the dots, and I start at the beginning with my story, and how this research started in the first place.

Chapter One

My Story

I began my research by trying to find the root cause of asthma, after watching my youngest son, at three years old, lie in a hospital bed with an oxygen mask, unable to breathe because of an asthma attack, and being told that the treatment wasn't working.

One of the senior doctors, a Registrar on ward round, said that his Consultant had tried a new method of delivering the nebulised drug over a longer period which had had some success in other patients. They tried it, and thank goodness it worked. I will be forever grateful to those doctors and nurses, and also to the pharmaceutical company for finding those drugs.

It left me feeling concerned though, as, although my eldest son and I also had mild asthma and had always been treated successfully by the drug salbutamol (Ventolin); for the first time in my life I saw that these drugs may not work, and so my journey to finding ways to prevent the asthma happening in the first place began. I wanted to know what was triggering the asthma, and, importantly, if I could find a way to prevent that happening.

My research, because of my eldest son having asthma, had already taught me that dust mites and being exposed to cow's milk in early life could trigger asthma. I couldn't go back in time to prevent what had happened to my sons, but I could remove some of these triggers by taking out carpets, get allergen-free bedding and vacuum and dust every day! Although research at the time did not link dairy products to asthma after the first months of life, I wanted to remove all known triggers out of my youngest son's diet as he had had such a bad episode. However, I was concerned about removing essential nutrients like calcium from his diet and so when I wanted to remove dairy from his diet I checked this with my Health Visitor. She said that there was plenty of calcium in broccoli, which my children ate and loved, and so didn't see a problem, and he became dairy free.

I also found that other things in a person's environment may be a trigger in some people, including some colours in foods, which were found in the sweets that my children ate, and so I became an avid ingredient reader! I should say here that I didn't give them sweets on a regular basis (and they both loved the small packets of raisins when they wanted something sweet) but one colour, at the time, had been banned in other countries as it affected brain development, and so my sons and I decided that it might be best to avoid these colours! I found sweets with natural colours and non-dairy ice cream, which my youngest son loved, and which my eldest son also ate as he wanted to support his brother. There were lots of treats available for them which they absolutely loved and so they didn't feel deprived. As a matter of interest, my youngest son is now six feet one, has strong healthy bones and teeth and has never needed a filling, so clearly he was eating enough calcium! However, both my sons continued to get occasional asthma (after getting a cold for example), even though it was no longer life threatening, but I had learned as much as I could on my own and was resigned to the fact that I had done as much as I could.

Then, three years later, a new BSc (Hons) degree in Human Medical Genetics at the University of Nottingham began, and, as I was still keen to see if I could find out more about asthma, I became a mature student when my sons were six and nine years old.

I learned that a family history of asthma, allergies and eczema suggested that we had the genes which made us susceptible to getting them, and the way this works is that those genes react strongly (more than in other people) to certain environmental triggers, like pollen and dust mite poo for example, and start an immune response against them. This immune response causes the inflammation of the airways and the lungs, in the case of asthma, which causes a tightening of those airways (bronchus and bronchi) which makes it difficult for us to breathe.

I had also learned that most genes which have such bad effects (like making it difficult to breathe and so potentially causing death) don't survive throughout time, because they reduce a person's fitness to survive, and reproduce, so my first thought was, 'why would we actually have the genes which made it difficult for us to breathe?!'

It turned out that these genes make an immune protein, an antibody, called Immunoglobulin E (IgE) (the type of antibody raised in 'allergic' responses) which reacts in a tough and extreme way to invaders, like parasites, which cause damage and severe harm. However, they were being triggered by things like pollen, dust mite poo (sorry!) and other triggers of asthma, hay-fever and eczema. The puzzle to scientists was why they reacted in this way. Clearly the pollen is a foreign substance entering our body, but it isn't exactly a threat to health like a parasite; so why call in the armed forces? It turned out that the answer may lay in our past.

I undertook specialist research at university and found a link between IgE and populations with a huge worm burden, as IgE recognises and destroys these worms and some other parasites. If a population suffered badly from worms and parasitic infections (which we all did in the past), then the genes we have now would have been beneficial, as they would have attacked and destroyed the parasites, which lived inside us eating nutrients from the food we ate, competing with us for those essential nutrients. In other words, the people with those genes, in the environment at that time, were healthier than those without them.

This explained why we still have those genes in a population, as the people with those genes were healthier and probably survived better than those without the genes; but why are those genes triggered in response to pollen and other harmless triggers, that are clearly not worms or other parasites? Although the results of my research were interesting, most of us in the western world don't have worms and so I didn't think too much about that at first, but then I learned about the **'Hygiene Hypothesis'**, where our environment (particularly in our home) is now so free of dirt, (and free of worms and parasites), that, although we are 'primed and ready' to attack worms, there are none to attack; and so our genes become almost 'trigger-happy' (or over-reactive) and our immune system starts to attack other invaders, like pollen. It is only a theory but it seemed like a possibility.

Another supporter of the 'too clean' theory came from **non-industrialised countries**, where exposure to dirt and parasites still exists, and asthma, allergies and indeed many other chronic inflammatory disorders are rarely seen. The theory is that this exposure is seen as 'normal' by the body, which deals with these potentially harmful invaders effectively; and as the body is no longer 'primed, with nothing to act upon, it doesn't react to non-harmful substances like pollen in the same extreme way. It stops being 'trigger-happy', firing un-necessarily.

Being very 'clean' also destroys many bacteria in our environment, including those that live with us, and research into our relationship with bacteria has revealed amazing information that impacts on our health; but not necessarily in a bad way! You can read more about this throughout the book, but it may explain one aspect of the hygiene hypothesis.

So the hygiene hypothesis may possibly explain why my sons and I reacted to things like pollen, and the drug salbutamol (Ventolin) certainly helped if we did get asthma; but even if that was the explanation I still needed to find a cure for the *cause*, rather than just treat the symptoms, even if medication did alleviate suffering. Surely preventing it happening in the first place was the gold standard?

Unfortunately, at the end of my degree in 1998, I had come to a halt, as no research could help me find a prevention at that time, and achieving the gold standard was not possible. **Until now** that is, and the reason I found this out was because of what happened to my mum last year.

My mum provides the trigger for me to continue research, and find preventable root causes of chronic disorders.

In June 2014 my 82 year old mum fell down some uneven steps and broke her arm in two places. Medications, including codeine, made her severely constipated, with dreadful pain; she was given an anti-depressant as a treatment for IBS which made her more anxious but did not help the IBS, and a side effect of some of the medication also caused a feeling of 'numbness' in her limbs. One evening as she stood up, in October, just as her broken arm was healing, her foot felt numb with 'pins and needles' and gave way, causing her to fall against her TV stand, damaging her back. She was in extreme pain and very low after all the recent events and the effects of her medication. She was also taking levothyroxine for an under-active thyroid.

As she lost weight, suffered more with her IBS and became depressed I decided to research around the subject, as the various doctors were either unable to offer a cure or gave medication which seemed to be making it worse (no offence intended, it was all they had to offer and gave it under approved guidelines). She was suffering from two, if not three, chronic disorders, (under-active thyroid, IBS and depression) and so I dedicated myself to research, to try and find the trigger (or triggers) that was causing her symptoms. I started with the gut, as she had IBS. My own doctor had given me 'Colofac' for the same problem many years earlier, telling me that it was a mild anti-spasmodic. It really helped me, and so I bought some for mum, and she stopped the anti-depressants prescribed for her for the same disorder. Within a few days they started to work and she started to feel a little better. At the same time, my research into codeine taught me that it doesn't actually stop pain, but alters the mind so that it doesn't care about the pain as much. It had some pretty grim side effects which seemed to explain the difference in the way my mum was thinking and behaving. Luckily, as she is an intelligent woman, she could see that mind altering drugs may not be the best thing to take! She stuck to paracetamol, and again, began, slowly, to feel a bit better, in spite of being in pain still. She didn't take Ibuprofen as the doctor had told her that it would irritate her stomach (she had suffered from stomach and duodenal ulcers a few years before), but rubbed a gel on painful areas.

[Ibuprofen is a non-steroidal anti-inflammatory drug, NSAID, which inhibit production of prostaglandins, which are chemicals in our bodies that enhance inflammatory effects. However, prostaglandins are also needed for other processes in the body, including digestion. This is why inhibition of prostaglandins by NSAIDs can cause indigestion and stomach and duodenal ulcers.]

A light at the end of the tunnel

In brief, my research led me to understand that **probiotics** may help her gut become more in balance, and that some things, like **glutamine** may also help to keep the gut lining healthy (and so she took both of these).

She also took **oregano** capsules, as it was possible that they may destroy 'bad' bacteria and also **liquorice root**, as this allegedly helps with depression. I researched any contra-indications of taking the supplements, and none applied to my mum, but to be on the safe side, she only took liquorice capsules three times a week as it may be a contraindication for people with heart problems (which she does not have).

I also gave her a copy of the **ABO Blood Type diet**. There wasn't any scientific evidence to approve this diet that I could find, but I had tried it for myself (I am Group A) and felt so energised by it; and, as it wasn't a crazy unhealthy limiting 'diet', but rather suggested that some things were more beneficial than others, and that a few things may not be great for you, I thought it might be worth a try (at least while she felt so bad). She agreed, and followed the recommendations, but wasn't rigidly following it though, but rather eating what she loved, while keeping it in mind. Her main concern was that she was also enjoying the food as she felt instinctively that not enjoying it meant she didn't digest it so well.

(There has been some recent research into the Blood Group Diet, and you can read more about this later in the book in chapter sixteen).

After a week, mum's IBS was under control, she had normal bowel movements and, after two weeks, her depression had also gone. She returned to being fit and healthy, no IBS, no constipation, not at all anxious, mentally alert, back to doing her complicated crosswords, back to a healthy weight and, she says, feeling better than she had felt for most of her life! Full of joy! At the same time, she read 'A New Earth' by Eckhart Tolle, which suggests that keeping your mind in the present moment can alleviate anxious and fearful thought.

As a scientist, I didn't think that I had found a miracle cure, as I am well aware that we are all unique, and react differently to different things, with our own unique set of genes but the staggering results in mum led me to wonder if any of these things might help other people that were also suffering with the same dreadful disorders.

At the same time as mum, I took all of the same supplements, as I wanted to be a healthy 'control' (albeit not very scientific as the numbers of participants were too small, but it was all I had) and to make sure I could detect any possible adverse effects, which I could mention to my poor sick mum. I wasn't expecting the difference in my own health, but I no longer got asthma, bloating, or even colds (in spite of being surrounded by sneezing individuals!). I felt great!! I thought 'there may be something in this!'

It seemed that the probiotics, together with a few changes in our diet, plus a few additional supplements, had revolutionised our health. Could it really be that simple? It certainly seemed that way, but in order to help others I needed more than anecdotal evidence from a sample of two, I needed proper scientific proof. As a scientist, nothing else would do. I knew that recommending something, even if it seemed to do no harm, and seemed to do some good, without evidence, would lead, quite rightly, to condemnation by others. I also knew that unless my research could be evidenced, it was merely my opinion, and why should anyone listen? Where was my authority? My law training taught me that! Why had these probiotics and other supplements seemingly helped us? Was it a placebo effect? I doubted that as I wasn't suffering from anything that my poor mum was suffering, and was only taking them to ascertain any potential harm rather than try to treat asthma or susceptibility to colds, both of which had miraculously improved! But my doubt wasn't enough. I needed proof.

Although I had looked at the impact genes had on health sixteen years previously, I needed to know if anything had changed and if there was any new information. So I started my current journey by going back to my university education, back to DNA. I didn't think that this could be the whole cause of chronic disorders, although I knew that genes made us susceptible to getting certain diseases; but I also knew that it was still the current medical thinking.

I wanted to see if any recent research proved otherwise, and my scientific and legal training gave me the ability to do so. At last, I had hope (albeit as a result of only two people in a study!) that there could be a cure or prevention of chronic disorders. I needed to join many more dots to complete the picture.

The one thing that my recent research had unfolded, was that inflammation was seen in all chronic disorders, and inflammation is created by immune cells. Immune cells are made by your genes and so was there a link to our genes and DNA after all?

Chapter Two

Your Genes, Your DNA and Your Long Term Health
(Key system One)

If you remember, in the forward I said that there are five key systems *in* your body that are major players in your long term health; and these are

- Your DNA
- Digestion
- Your immune system
- Your gut bacteria and
- Your brain

All of these interact with each other dynamically; responding to our environment and adjusting their responses in order to keep us healthy. We start with the first of those here.

The Human Genome Project had finished after I completed my degree, and so was there anything new that could provide me with an answer? It turned out the answer was YES! But not in the way you might think. What our recent knowledge about the genes in your DNA shows is just how LITTLE influence those genes have on your health, which means that your environment dictates your health in the main (and your environment also includes the food that you eat). You don't need to understand genes and DNA to read this book (which is as well because my description is brief to say the least!), but what you might be interested in is that your genes can be (temporarily) affected by environmental factors which can then result in chronic disorders. Note that I said temporarily. They *can* be changed, and quickly.

As I mentioned earlier, the current thinking in the medical profession is that some people, with particular genes that make them susceptible to particular disorders, then suffer from those particular chronic disorders; but, unluckily, there are no drugs to cure them (there are drugs to help the 'symptoms' of the disorders but not the cause of them and so they can't be prevented by pharmaceutical drugs).

We can't alter our DNA and so it seemed hopeless. That was also my thinking until last year when I resumed my research. BUT! For anyone with a chronic disorder, who has been told that it is because of your genes and you have to accept that and live with it, please take this on board **right now**...

- Having certain genes does not mean that you are destined to have a chronic disorder
- Genes only account for a 2% - 30% risk (approximately) of actually getting that disorder, which means that 70 – 98% is not down to your genes.
- You are in control!

A trigger or triggers in our environment (which includes the food and drink we consume) is by far the majority influence on outcome, and explains why, if you have two **identical twins** with **identical DNA**, one may get one (or more) chronic disorders, like hypothyroidism and rheumatoid arthritis, and the other one remains healthy. The environment of both, including diet and lifestyle, plays the **major** factor in deciding a person's health. **The good news is that we now know what those triggers can be!** You can find out about these throughout the book, and in the chapter on solutions.

So approximately 70 – 98% of your health can be influenced by *your* choices. You may have a genetic susceptibility, inherited from your family, but with the right choices you can have a healthy body, healthy weight, and a healthy mind. Also, please know that it is **never too late**. A study of people in their **seventies** and **eighties**, over twenty years, showed that, by making some of these changes, their mortality outcome (causes of death, for example by cancer, heart disease etc.) reduced by 40% - 60%. That also means of course that their health outcomes improved by 40% - 60%!

By making a few choices, you can remove the trigger(s) of your disorder. They don't even have to be huge or difficult choices. Some of the things you will be reading about in the book are so easy that anyone can do them!!

We can read about the triggers which may be causing your chronic disorder later in the book, but before that I wanted to find out if environmental triggers could actually affect your DNA, so what exactly is DNA and how does it work?

DNA

DNA is made up of sequences of four 'bases' Guanine, Cytosine, Thymine, and Adenine, commonly written in their short form of G C T and A. We get one strand of DNA from one parent and one strand from the other and the two strands are bound together, forming a double helix (a double spiral shape).

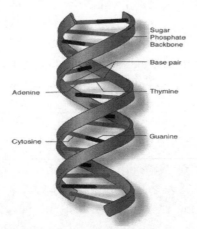

Image courtesy of the National Human Genome Research Institute's Talking Glossary (http://www.genome.gov/glossary/).

DNA is found in the chromosomes of every cell nucleus in (almost) every cell in the body, and is capable of making any product (we call all of these products 'proteins' usually) and any type of cell; for example an eye cell or kidney cell.

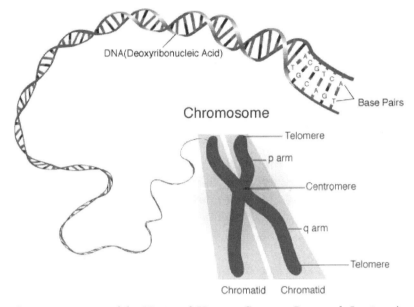

Image courtesy of the National Human Genome Research Institute's Talking Glossary (http://www.genome.gov/glossary/).

The DNA is capable of making these **proteins** because it is made up of **genes**, which carry instructions for *particular* proteins (for example ones needed to make a liver cell).

The rest is what we used to call 'junk' DNA, as it did not seem to have a function in the main; although some 'junk' DNA was known to control whether or not a particular gene is switched on or off. We now realise that even stretches of DNA a long way from a gene may still exert a huge influence on that gene. [*These bits of DNA may not be included in the transfer of new genes, or may be disrupted in the host DNA, in genetically modified products].*

All of the specific proteins from genes have different roles; for example some will become hormones, some will become cell structures and so on. Sometimes these complicated events go wrong and we get mutations, but we also have a security system, which recognises mistakes and gets rid of them (because these mutations can seriously damage your health, and can even lead to cancer).

In fact, we all get **cancer** cells, but our systems are so good at killing them off we never know about it! It is only when several of our defence security systems all go wrong together that we struggle to protect ourselves; but this can be prevented, and systems can heal if they are given a helping hand. Only ten percent of cancers have a genetic cause (and are seen in family members), but ninety percent of cancers are caused by environmental factors, like diet, lifestyle, alcohol and tobacco*.

*Ref: cancer research spokesperson on Dr Chatterjee programme

[If major genetic abnormalities occur, they exert a combination of major devastating effects. This is extremely rare though, and I only mention it for completeness].

Lock and Key

DNA is copied and replicated, repaired and replaced, mistakes cut out and replaced, and genes are expressed into specific proteins, which are then folded in a specific way to become active. The folding means that certain areas in different shapes are recognised elsewhere in the body, which are activated and cause a reaction onwards from there. It works like a 'lock and key'. In other words, you need the correct shaped key to unlock your door, and then you can open it and walk through. Try other shaped keys, it won't unlock and you can't walk through. These proteins have specific functions, like being a hormone or part of a muscle cell.

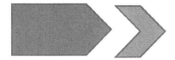

For those of you that are interested in reading more about genetics, there is a great website called GeneEd, which has talking lectures too. It can be found at http://geneed.nlm.nih.gov/index.php. If you are looking for a university to study it further, I can recommend the University of Nottingham!

Epigenetics – another layer of control

There has been some new and very exciting research in this area too, and the area of expanding research is in something called epigenetics, which means 'over genetics'. In other words, another layer of control, 'on top' of the information coded for by our genes. (For example, your genes have the information, the code, for your eye colour, but the additional epigenetic marker would switch off those eye colour genes in everywhere but your eyes).

Other types of differentiation also occur. For example some genes want to be active at certain times, for example when you are growing, but need to be silenced at other times, for example when you have stopped growing. This is a simple example but more complex systems still work on the same principle.

Epigenetics is the 'marking' of DNA with an extra layering of information (often by methylation, i.e. adding a methyl group) which adds additional instructions to the DNA. For example, the presence of a methyl group could determine whether the gene is active or silenced.

The whole system is extremely complicated, and other controls, such as tightly binding the DNA so that it can't be 'read', and systems, called imprinting, to ensure that only one strand of the DNA is read rather than both copies, exist, among others. An example of why these are necessary would be, if both mother's and father's genes are read and both genes make their proteins, we could have one parent's gene saying we have blue eyes and the other parent's gene saying they are brown. Where would we be?!

How 'junk' DNA can control your genes

The Human Gene Project, completed in 2003, discovered that the DNA of humans only contains around 22,000 genes. This was surprising because other (possibly more 'simple') life forms, can have more. For example, the Pinot grape has 30,000 genes! (*Source: Dr J. Bland, Functional Forum, March 2016*). In addition, most of the genes that humans *do* have are similar to primates; and so what makes us different? One part of the explanation is that our genes are read in 'families', and there are endless possibilities of forming different 'families' within those 22,000 genes, but things like anatomy, physiology, behaviour and intelligence could not be explained *only* by the DNA that is our *genes*.

So in **2003** the **National Human Genome Research Institute** (NHGRI) launched a public research project called **ENCODE** (Encyclopedia Of DNA Elements), to try and find out just what the 'junk' DNA contained, and if it had a function.

Breaking news

It turned out that junk DNA (which the project named 'dark matter'), does not produce proteins, but it does produce something called 'small RNA', which has an epigenetic influence on our genes, determining whether a gene is turned on or off, and controlling our development. It can also control the curling or uncurling of tightly bound DNA to allow genes to be 'read' or not. A surprising fact emerging from the research is that 88% of *disease*-causing mutations are found *outside* of genes, in the dark matter of the genome. The method of control comes from small molecular RNA, produced by the dark matter DNA, which folds, and then binds to DNA in your genes like a lock and key, in a similar way to that described above.

Even more extraordinary news was that dark matter *itself* is heavily influenced; and the surprising news is that **it is influenced by your diet, your environment and your lifestyle**; and these determine whether your *dark matter* is **activated** or not. In other words, **what you eat and how you live controls your genes**! So, to reduce cancer risk, chronic disorder risk; eat mainly vegetables, a little organic meat or wild fish if you wish to or eat vegetable protein like quinoa, nuts and beans; and, in addition, stay active, healthy, and stress-free, by taking regular exercise and meditation. You can find helpful ways to do this in the chapter on solutions.

One of the functions of dark matter is to produce the telomeres (ends) of chromosomes. When the DNA of a chromosome is replicated, the ends of the chromosome get shorter each time; until the chromosome cannot be replicated and the cell dies. This is the process of aging. However, with a nutritious diet, and healthy lifestyle, the aging process slows down, and so changing your diet, lifestyle and environment, as mentioned above, also keeps you looking younger!

The concept of changing our diet and lifestyle may not be too unfamiliar to us, but what about the links between thought and health? Four pioneering randomized control trials, including a total of 190 participants, looked at the effect of mindfulness meditation on telomeres. The result was that mindfulness meditation leads to a slowing down of telomere length reduction. Another study suggests that mindfulness can maintain telomere length in women who have survived breast cancer, possibly reducing cancer risk; although further studies are needed to confirm this.

Although many of us may fear being told that we have the BRCA 1 and 2 genes, which are linked to breast and ovarian cancer, these genes are actually tumour suppressor genes. The problem, if they mutate, is that they stop *preventing* the cancer, rather than be the cause of it.

How your genes are affected by food

The exciting new research provided a link between epigenetics, the environment and also *inherited* effects. We have known about epigenetics, and methylation, for a long time, but what has been learned fairly recently, is that environmental factors, such as a severe lack of food available to a mother during the first three months of pregnancy, can also be seen as an epigenetic marker on the DNA of her *grandchild*. In other words, an environmental factor, previously thought to only affect the person experiencing the effect (or her developing foetus), can be inherited! It is called the **Foetal Origins Hypothesis.**

The knowledge of environmental 'markers', like the lack of food, in themselves is not new, and studies on Drosophila fruit flies have shown how changes in the environment, during embryo development, can result in various mutations on the DNA of that embryo, like development of two pairs of wings; but it was thought that all such marking was removed in humans before the sperm and egg cells were made, and that the DNA was 'wiped clean' of this environmental information. It is this inheritability of environmentally-induced markers on DNA, that previously was not known to exist, which is having a major influence on our understanding of environmental factors on health. This epigenetic influence is not limited to the mother, as **paternal** epigenetic markers can also be inherited, influencing future generations.

Why would genes be marked in this way though? Well people who are best suited to their environment are the ones who will be most likely to reproduce and pass on their genes. One of the major impacts on survival is the type and availability of food sources, and how efficiently an individual can utilise those; and so the genes of the foetus are marked (an epigenetic marking called metabolic imprinting), which adapts those genes to the particular environment they are going to be born into.

For example, if food is scarce the genes of the foetus will be marked during a critical period of development, and this will affect the metabolic responses of the offspring, both inside and outside of the womb, to maximise all food sources that are available. In other words, the child is adapted to an environment with a scarcity of food. What was thought to be impossible however, is that not only the baby of a woman can be affected, but also the grandchild of that same woman. Metabolic imprinting is an inherited trait.

The way that this new knowledge was discovered in humans is as a result of natural environmental factors happening within a particular population; as, obviously, humans cannot and should not be experimented upon (some would say nor should animals but that is an ethical issue that would take a whole book in order to discuss it fully, so I won't expand on this here).

Such a natural event occurred for a group of people living through the Dutch famine of 1944–1945, and a study of hundreds of men and women showed that a poor maternal diet in early gestation was linked to increased obesity in middle-aged women at the age of 50 years. The men were not affected.

Another study that showed metabolic imprinting involved women living in Gambia, who eat seasonally available foods (sometimes in short supply at certain times of the year); which showed how certain food choices, and availability, affect their offspring, and even their grandchildren. Altered DNA methylation patterns could be seen in the offspring whose mothers were either exposed to famine or who conceived in the Gambian rainy season. As we mentioned above, it is sometimes referred to as the **'Foetal Origins Hypothesis'**.

In both the Dutch famine, and for the ladies of Gambia, where pregnant mothers were under-nourished, the offspring developed into obese adolescents, contrary to what was expected. It appears that a child being born into a harsh environment, where food is scarce, may have epigenetic markers which adapt it to making the most of available nutrients. However, in times of plenty, these markers actually cause the child to become obese, if the environment has changed.

In summary

Our genes interact with our environment, on a continual basis, adapting to external conditions, such as food availability or temperature. This interaction allows humans to develop, adapt and survive. Your genes, your diet, your lifestyle, and your thoughts, all interact, dynamically 'talking' to one another with chemical signals. This can result in either health or disease, but neither are set, and many are reversible.

For example, the protein galanin regulates appetite, among other things, and is produced in the brain. An over-production of galanin not only affects the size of someone's appetite but it also influences their food choices. For example, someone may have a preference for fatty food or alcohol. The bit of DNA that controls the genes which produce galanin is in the dark matter DNA; and it tells the genes where, when and how much protein to produce; BUT, if we eat/drink nutritious food, this may alter the production of galanin in our body. Galanin is a neuropeptide, which is linked to a number of chronic disorders including **Alzheimer's disease, epilepsy, depression,** and **cancer**; and so we can see how a simple change in our diet and lifestyle may protect us from chronic disorders which were thought to be untreatable.

Breaking news

Even more recent research indicates that brain disorders like autism may be caused by epigenetic marking of our DNA, and these epigenetic changes are potentially reversible. As we just read, nutrition and the avoidance of potential triggers are extremely important factors, and can explain why identical twins do not necessarily get the same chronic disorders, such as cancer or type 2 diabetes. We talk about solutions for these later in the book in chapter thirteen.

Junk DNA and environmental stress

Other environmental influences, like the **'ice storm babies'** in Canada can also be seen as epigenetic marking in our DNA. In the ice storms of January 1998, more than 3 million people in Quebec were without heating and light for almost 45 days and the temperatures plummeted. A team followed a group of about 150 families, in which the mother was pregnant during the ice storm or became pregnant shortly afterwards, to see if it affected the unborn children. In June 2014, when the children were teenagers, the team showed links between the ice stress and the development of symptoms of **asthma** and **autism** in the children; and that the children had distinct epigenetic methylation on their DNA.

Take home message

- We are more than the DNA that makes proteins (our genes).
- The thing that differentiates human DNA from plants and other animals is the large amount of 'junk' DNA that humans have.
- Junk DNA is now called dark matter, and it is where life is regulated

- The major factors affecting your dark matter are your diet, environmental factors, your lifestyle and your wellbeing.

The final point to remember here is not to be alarmed. Epigenetics is a constantly shifting marker on your DNA, which you can change with a few simple adjustments to your life. The chapter on solutions tells us how to do this.

Our health system, to date, has focused on trying to find risk and causes of disease. Diagnosis. However, most of your DNA does not code for disease, but for wellness; and so, taking an alternative view of genetic testing, we could use testing not to diagnose disease but to increase our ability to be well. We need to look forwards, with prognosis, and not backwards, with diagnosis (my opinion).

HLA Genes

We all have a group of genes called the HLA (human leucocyte antigen) complex; more than 200 genes located close together on chromosome 6. It is the HLA that determines which cells are 'you' and which ones are 'foreign. It also determines which bacteria we tolerate in our gut and which we destroy; and this partly explains why we see a diversity of strains of particular commensal bacteria between different humans, as we all have a unique HLA genes, allowing each person's immune system to react to a wide range of foreign invaders.

More than 100 diseases have been associated with different variations of the HLA genes, and these include autoimmune diseases such as type 1 diabetes, Hashimoto thyroiditis and rheumatoid arthritis.

However, as we just read, having genes which make you susceptible to getting a disorder does not mean that you will get it, and we can read more about this in the chapter on solutions.

DNA and your gut.

Some other research which links to this new information about diet, epigenetics, and another layer of control on top of your DNA, comes not from *outside* of your body, but from what lies *within*! To be more precise, from the microbes that live in your gut, and you can read more about this exciting new research in chapter five; but before we do, it is important to understand that **nothing in your body acts in isolation**. Your **digestive tract** and the way it works, your **immune system** (much of which lies just below your intestines), your **brain** and your **gut microbes** are **all** linked; to each other, to other systems in your body and to chronic disorders. We know that the digestive system and immune systems are closely linked to chronic and autoimmune disorders, so let us remind ourselves (briefly!) how the digestive system works, then how immune cells in the digestive tract work, and how these might contribute to your chronic disorder. After that, we can read about the exciting new research about the microbes that live in your digestive tract.

Take home message:

- We have genes which make us susceptible to getting certain specific disorders. BUT!
- There is a second level of control, on top of our genes, which means that the genes can be controlled by things in our environment, such as our diet and lifestyle. This is called epigenetics.
- It is now known that epigenetic markers are also able to be inherited. BUT!
- As each individual's chosen environment also affects their health outcome, then having certain susceptibility genes, or even inherited epigenetic markers, doesn't mean that we have a problem! The chapter on solutions tells us more.

Chapter Three

Digestion and Your Long Term Health
(Key System Two)

It was thought, for many years, that the digestive tract, running from mouth to anus, was a fairly simple 'tube', in which we break down, digest, and absorb nutrients from the food that we eat. Recent research has completely changed those thoughts, but before I explain why, I will give a brief and simplified explanation of the digestive tract.

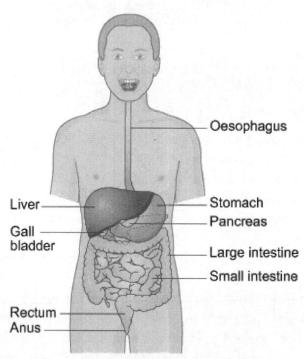

Oesophagus

Liver

Stomach

Pancreas

Gall bladder

Large intestine

Small intestine

Rectum
Anus

Mouth - digestion begins here, where your teeth break down large chunks into smaller bites, and digestive enzymes in saliva (chemicals made by the body) begin to break down the food even further (starches start to be broken down into sugars here). The food is swallowed and moves on to the

Stomach - which produces further digestive enzymes like pepsin, which breaks down large proteins into smaller peptides.

O-O-O-O-O-O-O   →   O-O-O   O-O-O-O

Proteins   Peptides

Proteins are made of combinations of twenty different amino acids, shown here as circles O O O .

We can make eleven of them, but we need to get the other nine from our food, so these nine amino acids are called 'essential' amino acids. There are also ones called 'conditional' amino acids, which we don't normally need because we can make them, but may need in times of stress or illness; and these include **glutamine**, which can be taken as a supplement. Proteins can be hundreds of amino acids long, and the amino acids join together to give the protein its unique 'lock and key' shape.

The stomach also contains hydrochloric acid (HCl), which kills off many pathogenic (harmful) microbes and aids digestion (particularly of meat). The stomach also stores the food until the small intestine is ready to receive it, as you can eat a meal faster than your intestines can digest it.

29

Some foods and liquids (like alcohol) are absorbed through the lining of the stomach, but the majority pass to the

Small intestine – where the muscles in the wall of the intestines mix your food with even more enzymes produced there (and also move food along towards the end of the gut). Enzymes made by the pancreas (trypsin and others) enter the small intestines and these are needed to break down and digest food. Here, for example, peptides are broken down into the building blocks of proteins, found in all living things, the amino acids. Amino acids, glucose molecules and fatty acids (the end result of digestion of food) pass through the small intestine epithelium into the bloodstream below, where they are taken to the liver and then on to other cells in the body.

Your DNA uses the amino acids to make the unique proteins (like muscle cells and hormones for example) needed for your body; glucose is used for energy, and fatty acids are used to make hormones, among other things (in simple terms).

[The pancreas is also part of our endocrine system, and secretes a hormone, insulin, into the bloodstream when blood sugar levels rise. It is essential for keeping blood sugar levels within normal ranges (not too high or too low).

Insulin allows the glucose to be taken into the cells of your body where it is used in cellular respiration (to make energy). It also allows this soluble glucose to be converted to an insoluble carbohydrate called glycogen which is stored in your liver and muscles.]

The small intestine also has a special feature, in that it has a huge surface area, created by millions of **villi**, which are tiny finger-like structures with small blood vessels inside. This large surface area helps to increase the amount of nutrients absorbed by the body. The villi have even more hair like structures, called **microvilli**, on their surface, providing an even more massive surface area, the size of a football pitch, to aid efficient absorption of nutrients.

The lining of the intestines (the epithelium) is only one cell thick, and this allows the tiny nutrients released by digestion of food (amino acids from proteins, fatty acids from fats and glucose from carbohydrates) to pass through them and enter the blood. The cells in the epithelium were thought to be 'cemented' together, but it is now known that they are linked by **Tight Junctions**, which normally remain closed.

There is also a mucous layer which protects the gut lining, and separates the gut contents from the **immune cells,** and blood vessels, which lie below the mucous layer. Most of the important nutrients, the end products of digested food, like amino acids and glucose, needed by the body, are absorbed at different points along the small intestine into the bloodstream. These nutrients are the same in all life forms and so do not invoke an immune response when they enter the blood stream. However, in addition to this, any potential immune trigger which may have remained on these tiny nutrients is removed.

Another important point to note is that anything in the digestive system is still technically 'outside of the body'. Only when things pass out of the digestive tract do they 'enter the (rest of your) body. Any food which *does* invoke an immune response must have come into contact with immune cells lying beneath the gut mucosal layer. This should not happen as food any bigger than its component parts (like amino acids from protein) is too big to pass through the gut lining; and so implies that the gut has become leaky in some way. There has been some exciting research into this and we talk about this more in chapter nine.

Food that can't be digested and absorbed by the small intestine (like the soluble and insoluble fibre from plants) pass into the

Large intestine – which absorbs water from the remains of the food which was digested, and absorbed, in your small intestine. Bacteria and other microbes in the large intestine also help with the final stages of digestion, and we talk about these more in chapters five and six. Although the large intestine is divided into different areas, one of those areas, the

Colon - is where the vast majority of your commensal bacteria actually live (called commensal because they can live in our body without doing us harm and we also help them, unlike pathogenic bacteria, which are harmful). Other microbes, like yeasts and some viruses also live in the colon. These microbes live in the mucosal layer of your gut and attach themselves to your gut lining. Collectively these bacteria and other microbes are called the **microbiome.** Although some microbes live in the last part of the *small* intestine, where the small and large intestines meet, in general they are not tolerated in the small intestine and are destroyed (it makes sense, as this is where you absorb your nutrients, and so they would be competing with you for food!)

All of the nutrients you need have now been absorbed out of your small intestine and into your bloodstream, but you cannot utilise fibre from plants, and so this passes into the colon, with other waste. This is great news for the bacteria in your colon which can and do digest the *soluble* fibre in the fruit and vegetables, living very happily on it and thriving well. This is one of the reasons why we can all live happily with these bacteria, as they do not eat our food and we provide them with the food they need! The insoluble fibre (the cell walls of the fruit and vegetables) also plays an important role in gut health, and helps in gut motility (movement) and is also needed to bulk up the stool. The microbiome was not considered to play a particularly important role until recently, but new research has shown that your gut microbes play an *essential* part in your life. I explain more about this in chapter six

Once the remains of your food has been in the large intestine for 3-10 hours it becomes semi-solid because most of the water has been removed. These remnants, of dead bacteria from both your food and colon, and undigested food, get passed out of the body as faeces.

What happens when we eat more than we need?

We have two hormones which tell us that we are hungry (ghrelin) and full (leptin); but sometimes we override leptin!

When you eat food, your body converts it to its constituent parts, like amino acids, fatty acids and glucose, which are passed from your gut into your bloodstream, and these are then used by your body to make proteins, repair your body where necessary, and for energy (in simple terms).

Eating an *excess* of food is something our bodies have adapted to over hundreds of years, and the available energy from that food is stored in the form of fat stores in the body, and glycogen in the liver and muscles, so that we have an energy source for when food is less plentiful. Most human fat is found directly beneath the skin and is called adipose tissue, although some is also stored around your organs.

Why is digestion a key system?

One of the reasons we get chronic and autoimmune disorders is because our bodies become bombarded with things that trigger the disorders, and this can include some of the foods that we eat and digest. To find any food triggers that you may have, the elimination diet, found later in the book, is the gold standard. Another reason why we may get chronic disorders is not because of what we eat but because of what we don't eat. Again, the food that is optimal for your health can be found later in the book, in the elimination diet and also in the chapter on solutions.

As we just read, as well as feeding human cells in our body, what you eat also feeds the microbes that live in your gut, but does this matter and do the food choices that you make affect these microbes? The answer to both of those is yes, and I will explain why in chapters five and six. However, before we explore more about our amazing gut bacteria, and how they keep us healthy, I needed to know why our immune system doesn't kill off the bacteria that live in our gut! How can we have a foreign invader living with us in the first place?!

Take home message

- Your food is broken down, throughout our digestive system, into smaller and smaller pieces, eventually into its component parts (like breaking down protein into amino acids for example) which are then absorbed by your body from the small intestine.

- Your intestines have a lining (the epithelium) which is only one cell thick. This is impermeable to large particles and so only tiny nutrients, like amino acids, can pass through. The cells in your small intestine are joined together in places by Tight Junctions, and these normally remain closed. Some triggers can cause these Tight Junctions to open (explained later in the book).

- Your small intestine also houses a major part of your immune system, which lies below the mucous layer lining your intestines, separating your gut contents from your immune cells, which lie below the mucous layer. Any food which does invoke an immune response must have come into contact with immune cells lying beneath the gut mucosal layer. This should not happen as food any bigger than its component parts (like amino acids from protein) is too big to pass through the gut lining; and so implies that the gut has become leaky in some way. There has been some exciting research into this (see chapter nine).

- Your colon houses your microbiome, which thrives on the soluble fibre in your food (vegetables and fruit) which you cannot digest.
- All of your digestive tract is protected by a layer of mucous, made by the cells of the digestive tract.

Chapter Four

Your Immune System (briefly!) and Your Long Term Health (Key System Three)

Our immune system is one of the 'dots' of information I joined that gave me the overall picture of how chronic and autoimmune disorders develop, and I researched it for two reasons. One is that I wanted to know why our immune system doesn't kill off the bacteria living in our gut, and the second is because all chronic disorders (those that last longer than three months) have chronic inflammation, as a result of an activated immune system, and I wanted to find out why.

[Your doctor will tell you that many long term chronic disorders cannot be cured, because they are a problem of your immune system. While they *are* a problem involving your immune system, what doctors mean is that there is no *pharmaceutical* cure, and that is true; but that doesn't mean that there is no cure at all. Your doctor may not be able to provide you with medication to make you better, but you no longer have to accept that there is no cure for your long term health problems.]

So here is a very simple explanation of our immune system!

All living things have a cluster of genes called the MHC genes (called HLA genes in humans), that have a unique gene-shuffling process which makes millions of different immune cells, each with a unique recognition pattern on their surface, which allow our immune cells to recognize millions of potential pathogens that it comes into contact with.

All the immune cells which recognise 'self' are destroyed in your thymus before they are allowed to enter your blood circulation, to avoid them attacking your own body. At least, that was the thinking until 2015, when breaking research discovered that the cells (called T cells) which recognise 'you' are not destroyed but they very rarely, if ever, respond. That is, under normal circumstances.

However, if those immune cells come into contact with something that isn't normally found in your bloodstream, something that is an 'invader' but is also very similar to 'your' proteins, then they *may* become active. An example of food proteins that are similar to human proteins can be seen in both wheat (similar to the cells of the gut lining) and milk (some proteins are similar to the thyroid gland). We call this 'molecular mimicry'. My opinion is that our normally inactive immune 'self' T-cells may be activated if these food proteins find their way into our bloodstream. Normally that would never happen, as they are too big to pass through the intestine wall (and food proteins do not invade us like a bacteria can!) but new research has discovered that our intestines can sometimes be 'leaky', and I talk more about this in chapter nine

The immune cells mature into different types. Some float freely in the blood and engulf anything that they encounter which is not 'you', and go to the nearest lymph gland to 'present the invader'. If the invader is harmless, like pollen, it is destroyed and eliminated from your body. These simple 'detect and destroy' immune cells, like macrophages, are called the **innate immune system.** Some innate immune cells are also found in tissues. However, you have *two* sorts of immune systems, and these are called the **'innate' immune system** and the **'acquired' immune system'**

Your **acquired immune system** comes into play if the invading particle (which your innate immune cells have taken to the lymph gland) is recognised by the 'pattern' on one of your immune cells, as being an invading bacteria or virus. The acquired immune system consists of **B cells**, which make antibodies (also called immunoglobulins, like IgA, IgG and so on) against the *specific* bacteria or virus which your innate immune cells found, and two types of **T cells** (so called because they come from the thymus).

One type of T cell, the **T-helper** cell is the main regulator of your immune responses, and it becomes activated *only if* it recognises the invader. Once activated, the **T-helper** cells make messenger proteins which activate other immune cells, including the **B cell** that located the specific invading bacteria in the first place.

This then causes that particular B cell to make lots of duplicate copies of *itself* (called antibodies, or immunoglobulins), which then attack the *specific* invader (like a flu virus for example). Your immune system is super quick and efficient, and can make thousands of specific antibodies in seconds.

The other type of T cell are **T killer cells**, and these have receptors that they use to search each cell that they meet. If the cell is infected with a virus, it is quickly killed. The infected cells are recognized because tiny traces of the intruder can be found on their surface.

The proteins which T cells make, in order to activate other immune cells are called **cytokines,** and these act as 'messengers' from one immune cell to another.

Cytokines are made by many different cells but the main producers are T-helper cells and macrophages.

Some cytokines are *pro*-inflammatory, creating inflammation, whereas others are *anti*-inflammatory and reduce inflammation.

Both the innate and acquired immune cells can trigger inflammation, and, together, they have several important functions:

> 1. The inflammation isolates the invading bacteria or viruses, protecting the rest of the body from invasion and also

protecting the damaged area, creating a 'cushion' which prevents further harm and which creates an area within which damaged cells can be taken away and new healthy cells can be brought to replace them. Damage gone, repairs made, healthy cells restored, all rubbish taken away. As we do in our external environment, we need to clear out the rubbish to stay healthy.

2. The immune cells also release chemicals which trigger increased permeability of local capillary walls to allow the large immune cells to escape from the constraints of the blood vessels and get into the tissues, to the source of the 'non-self' invader, to kill and destroy them. This influx of blood into the tissues is why we get the redness, heat and localised swelling that we see and feel. The killed invaders are taken away with damaged cells as described above. This swelling also presses on local nerves, which gives you the feeling of pain, but is part of the healing process.

One of these inflammatory responses is seen in 'hay-fever' sufferers; where mucous linings in the airways swell and noses run. The inflammation is caused by mast cells (part of our innate immune system) which make and release histamine.

[*The most common treatment for these seasonal allergies is 'anti-histamine', which stops the inflammation and histamine production, relieving the symptoms. Of course, this immune response by the mast cells would be useful if the invader was a harmful invader like a cold virus!*].

Note however that this anti-histamine 'treatment' is for the prevention of the 'symptoms' (the swelling and increased fluid associated with the inflammation and removal of the invading cell) and does *not* treat the *root cause*.

Why is the immune system a key system?

We now know that chronic disorders all share chronic inflammation as a common factor, (no matter what name the disorder or disease is given), and the reason we have this is because our immune system is continually trying to repair some sort of ongoing damage, or respond to an ongoing trigger, and this response brings with it ongoing inflammation, with associated pain.

Let me just say here that inflammation is not a bad thing *per se*. In fact it is usually a good thing, as any damaged areas of the body are protected with a cushion of inflammation while the damage is being repaired. This is acute inflammation, resulting from either normal cell replacement or because of some sort of damage signal, due to invasion or physical trauma, and is a short term measure. The difference between acute inflammation and chronic inflammation is that acute inflammation goes when the damage or trigger goes, whereas chronic inflammation does not stop, which is why it is called 'chronic' inflammation.

How does pain relief work?

The drugs given to 'treat' most chronic disorders (or rather the chronic inflammation symptoms of them which happen as a result of an immune response) are anti-inflammatory drugs (like Ibuprofen) called NSAIDs (non-steroidal anti-inflammatory drugs), which are given to stop the inflammation as their title suggests!

Why anti-inflammatory drugs? Well as we read earlier in this chapter, inflammation results in an increased pressure on surrounding nerves which causes pain signals to go to the brain. For example, in the case of rheumatoid arthritis, inflammation occurs at the joints because this is where the damage occurs and, as we read earlier, our body creates inflammation to protect the damaged area and allows the body a cushion in which it can repair the damage. However, as the swelling isn't normally there we feel the pressure of it on nearby nerves, which then send a 'pain' signal to the brain. (This is a very simple summary and it can be complex).

If NSAIDs treat the symptoms why not just keep taking them?

I considered that too, but another reason for writing this book is that I also learned from my research that the anti-inflammatory drugs either become ineffective over time or make the condition worse! Now that was a shock!! Another reason why I decided to write this book!

It isn't difficult to see why the patient feels 'better' after taking the drugs, as the swelling is reduced and so the pain has gone, but it is also easy to see how further damage, for example to the joints, can occur without the protective aspect of the inflammation, which also allows, and is in fact essential for, healing and repair. I suspect that most patients aren't aware that their 'treatment' is only to remove the pain symptoms and is not in fact treating the underlying cause. I liken it to seeing a warning light in your car indicating that your engine is overheating, stopping the car, getting out, cutting the wire to the light, and starting to drive again. You can't see the warning light anymore but you can be sure that the overheating in the engine hasn't gone away and will probably get much worse!

It is for these two reasons, the ineffectiveness of drugs to treat chronic disorders and the potential harm caused by the drugs given to treat the *symptoms* of chronic disorders, together with an event which happened to my mum (see chapter 1) that led me to finally decide to write this book.

Taking control of your health

As the 'treatment' really looked at the smoke and not the fire, and as lots of really good research might not be put into practice for years, I felt that it would be useful for people to know about some of that excellent research right now, allowing them to make positive changes to their health outcomes, all under their own control. Taking medication which treats only the symptoms, is like taking pain medication because you have a drawing pin stuck in your foot. The drawing pin is the problem and that is what this book can help you find. The root cause.

Before I continue, I'd like to repeat that there are endless studies which suggest that many chronic disorders can be prevented and, in many cases, be reversed, so don't despair!

Also, it is worth repeating here that it is never too late. A study of **people in their seventies** and **eighties**, over twenty years, showed that, by making some of these changes, their mortality outcome (causes of death, for example by cancer, heart disease etc.) reduced by 40% - 60%. That also means of course that **their health outcomes improved by 40% - 60%!**

A final point to make here is that most pharmaceutical drugs come with side effects, whereas the changes that you make will be free of those. I should say here that the drugs I mentioned are the anti-inflammatory drugs, which may be extremely helpful to remove pain in the short term, but *some* drugs do much more than that, and are *essential* and do an amazing job. For example, insulin, if you need to take it, saves lives, and the drug for Hashimoto's thyroiditis (levothyroxine) is also a wonderful drug which is essential for your body if your thyroid gland is not working properly; and so I don't criticise drugs *per se*, as some, like these, are essential, and others can offer pain relief when it becomes unbearable. **This book isn't about stopping your drugs today and embarking on a new regime, but working together with your doctor to hopefully reduce the drugs that you need and, in some cases, prevent the need for you to have to take them at all! A new approach.**

Take home message

- You have an innate and acquired immune system, which 'talk' to each other via messengers called cytokines.
- Cytokines can either cause or stop inflammation.
- Inflammation is created by your immune cells in response to damage or an invader.
- Acute inflammation is short term, and stops as soon as the damage heals or the invader is destroyed.
- Chronic inflammation is ongoing, because the damage, trigger or invader persist in the body.
- Your immune cells only detect invaders, or indicators of their presence, which are in the bloodstream, either by meeting the whole cell, or meeting up with indicators of damage, like bits of DNA (which are only normally found within a cell).
- Some drugs for chronic disorders reduce pain, and others are essential; needed to save your life and help your body to function normally

Before we leave the chapter on the immune system, I still had one question that had not been answered: Why doesn't our immune system kill off the bacteria in our gut? To answer this, we need to take a closer look at our gut microbiome (not literally you will be pleased to know!!), in the next chapter.

Chapter Five

The Gut Microbiome and Your Long Term Health
(Key system Four)

[Collectively the gut (colon) bacteria, plus other microbes, in our body are called the microbiota, and their collective DNA is called the microbiome. These two terms are interchangeable, but the one most commonly used is the microbiome and so this is the term I use in this book.]

Why is the gut microbiome a key system?

The gut microbiome consists of a complex community of microbe species that live in your digestive tract. Some microbes are found throughout your digestive tract but the vast majority live in the part of your large intestine called the colon. Your relationship with these microbes is commensal and symbiotic (you need them and they need you). The exciting breaking news is that your gut microbiome does more than just 'eat' the fibre you don't digest, as it also has an **enormous effect on your health**

As we have already mentioned, it was once thought that the gut comprises a complex 'hosepipe', which starts at the mouth and ends at the anus. Its function, it was thought, was to take in food, which was then systematically digested into smaller particles until these were absorbed into the rest of the body outside of the intestines. These particles, like amino acids and glucose, are then utilised by your body to make things like proteins, with various functions, and to give you energy (in simple terms). A fairly simple process, it was thought, involving digestive enzymes, some hormones, some acid (in the stomach) and a ripple movement, called peristalsis, to keep the food moving along in the right direction. We knew that we tolerated some bacteria which inhabited the gut, but their function, if any, was not well known. **Until now.**

More recent studies have found that your gut bacteria play a huge role in your physical and mental health. I will explain more about that in this chapter, but before I do I just said that nutrients were passed out of your intestines into 'the rest of your body'. This has special significance, as the gut acts almost like an 'external' feature of our body, much like the skin; and both the skin, and the gut, protect us from potentially harmful 'invaders'. They do this in two ways. The first is to provide a tight barrier to the outside world, and the second is that we are protected by the bacteria which live on our surfaces.

We tend to think of all **bacteria** as being 'bad' and 'harmful', but that isn't necessarily the case. There are harmful bacteria of course, and not many of us underestimate the dangers that bacteria can pose. For example, disease caused by some species of gut bacteria is the leading cause of death in the world, with **Shigellosis** alone causing over a million deaths a year. However, trillions of bacteria live in our gut without causing us harm, so we know that we can live together happily, but what we have underestimated is the full extent of how bacteria affect us, and how they do this. What is perhaps even more surprising to learn is that, not only are some bacteria *beneficial* to us, some bacteria, and other microbes, are actually *essential* for our health and wellbeing.

Bacterial cells outnumber human cells!

I first started to fully understand our relationship with bacteria when I was a student of human medical genetics from 1995 - 1998, I was amazed to learn from our professor that there were three times more bacterial cells on our body than human cells! They live on all surfaces that are exposed to the outside world, including your skin. We can't see them on our body, (which is probably as well), but before you feel totally creeped out by this fact, let me tell you the good news. We need these microbes. They keep us well and healthy. They are, simply, our closest friend!

Clearly we can live together, and we can tolerate their presence, but what we didn't know at the time of my degree was just how much *influence* these bacteria had on us. In fact, **the bacteria in our gut are essential for health**, and **without them we would not survive**. Another amazing new piece of knowledge is that although there are three times as many bacterial cells as human cells on our body as a whole, **there are actually ten times as many bacterial cells as human cells in our gut**; about 100 trillion in number, and these are critical to your health. It isn't really surprising that most of our commensal microbes are found in the gut, as most potentially harmful microbes are ingested, and our gut bacteria protect us from them. We need all the protection we can get. But how do bacteria protect us? I needed to understand more about our relationship with our gut bacteria, and, particularly, why we do not kill them off.

Why doesn't our immune system kill off the gut bacteria?

There has been a co-evolution of humans and bacteria over many years, and one part of this evolution might be seen in another important feature of the intestines, which is the mucous layer which lines it. This mucous layer in the colon houses our commensal microbes and a large percentage of our own immune system. It is almost like a daily battlefield where friends (commensal gut microbes) and enemies (pathogenic (disease-causing) microbes) must all be recognized by our immune cells in order to determine which of these microbes we will tolerate and which we need to destroy by initiating an immune response against them.

But *none* of these microbes are 'self', not even those that we call commensal (living in harmony with us), so why doesn't our immune system just attack and destroy *all* of these 'non-self' microbes? After all, that is what they are designed to do isn't it? In other words, how do we recognise and tolerate these foreign bacterial cells in the first place? It seemed that glycans may be the answer.

We read earlier in the book, in the chapter on the immune system, that your immune cells can recognise other cells, and they do this with glycans, which are complex sugar molecules (polysaccharides), covering the cell surfaces of immune cells. They also cover every cell in the body that faces the outside world, called **epithelial cells**, and they all recognise both other cells and various chemical signals like cytokines.

These glycans are found on the surface of our **immune** cells at specific sites, and recognise '**danger-associated molecular patterns**' or '**self-associated molecular patterns**' of glycans on the cells which they interact with. Glycans are also found on some bacteria, and are called Lipopolysaccharides (LPS).

It is also these glycans that microbes attach to in order to invade us, and so it is a double edged sword, and a constant battle between the two! (Sometimes, invading bacteria hi-jack the pattern of glycans on our epithelial cell surfaces, in order to disguise themselves as being human. Humans combat this by adding additional random patterns of glycans onto their cell surface, in order to find the 'foreign' bit of the invading bacterial cells).

However, the way that the commensal bacteria may communicate with human cells when they inoculate the foetus may also be via these glycans.

So that may explain how our body recognises 'self' and 'non-self', via glycans, but it doesn't explain why we don't destroy the commensal bacteria, which are, after all, not 'self'. There has been much research on this subject, but as bacteria interact with their host, it isn't always easy to determine this interaction outside of the body. However, the initial microbial colonization of babies, originally thought to occur in the first few months of a baby's life, but now thought to happen in utero, coincides with both the *functional* maturation and also the *structural* maturation of the human intestinal immune system. As the immune system is not yet developed, the presence of the microbes in the baby results in regulation of the very immune response that would destroy them. However, not only are these microbes tolerated, because they appear to invade prior to an established immune system, they appear to play an important role in the *development* of that immune system, early in infancy.

In fact, many studies seem to indicate that those first intestinal microbes to inhabit a baby provide an essential stimulus to the maturation of both the actual physical gut and that of the immune system there (reviewed by Hooper).

One thing that is well established is that bacterial **lipo-polysaccharides (LPS)** (also known as 'lipo-glycans' and 'endotoxin'), which are found on their cell surface, have been conserved throughout time, and it is these stretches of conserved structure on the surface of the bacterial cells (the lipo- 'glycans') that are recognised by our immune cells (by the 'glycans' on our immune cell surface). The actual recognition of the pattern of these different glycans is by something called Toll-like Receptors (TLRs).

These TLRs recognise the LPS (bacterial glycans) of both commensal and pathogenic bacteria and they play a crucial role in host defence against infection by these bacteria.

I was still confused. I could see how the commensal bacteria might get into a human in the first place, but I still didn't understand why they aren't eventually recognised and destroyed by a human's mature immune system. Why aren't those conserved regions of the bacterial lipo-glycans (LPS) recognised as foreign and destroyed?

The answer may lie in the fact that the conserved regions on the LPS are *specific* to certain *types* of bacteria, and so some types of gut bacteria (the ones that colonise a human early in life) may not be recognised as an 'enemy' if they co-evolved with humans. In fact, as we mentioned, it is thought that the recognition of these particular commensal bacteria by the Toll-like Receptors 'teach' a new immune system, and so are critical for defence against pathogens. This relationship between TLRs and commensal bacteria only remains in balance while the gut is not damaged and the bacteria do not stray out of the gut and into the bloodstream. In this instance, if our immune system detects these commensal bacteria in the blood stream instead of them being nicely contained in the gut, the immune system then becomes activated to attack the bacteria.

Bacteria can exert an epigenetic control over your genes

If you remember from the chapter on our DNA, there is another layer of control on top of the DNA called epigenetics, which modifies the genes in some way (for example to be switched on or off where needed) usually by methylation (adding a methyl group marker to the DNA). Commensal bacteria have utilised this epigenetic process of modification, and are actually able to control the gene that makes the Toll-like Receptors (which, in turn, recognise the bacteria that normally initiate an immune attack against them). The gene is called the TLR4 gene. But how do they do this?

- *Recent studies show that commensal bacteria can control the epigenetic modification of the human TLR4 gene in the large intestine by epigenetic methylation.*

Methylation of the human TLR4 gene causes it to become down-regulated, and so much less responsive to the bacterial lipo-glycans which, as we have just read, have 'patterns', or 'shapes', that our immune cells recognise as foreign. Because of this modification of the TLR4 gene, our immune cells still recognise the bacteria, but this down-regulation quietens any excessive immune response.

Interestingly, TLR4 genes are found in all life, from Drosophila fruit flies to humans, and they play a fundamental role in pathogen recognition in us all. In humans this pathogen recognition (which is actually just recognition of 'non-self') also leads to activation of the innate immune cells, and production of cytokines (which are messengers to instruct other immune cells to come to the area to help attack and destroy the invader. Examples of cytokines are tumour necrosis factor and interleukins).

- *So to summarise, commensal bacteria can influence expression of our genes and immune response in the gut; and it is this control which causes our intestine's cell lining to be relatively unreactive to the trillions of commensal bacteria it is exposed to, and so not trigger an immune response against the microbiome as would happen with any other invader. Your microbiome is able to do this because it can exert an epigenetic control over your DNA (well, the DNA of specific genes like the TLR4 gene).*

Only if these microbes *become* harmful, and immune cells detect damage, does your immune system react against them. I said the intestines, but most of your microbes actually live in your colon, and survive on the soluble plant fibre that we can't digest as we already mentioned, and so they aren't in competition with us for nutrients we absorb via our small intestine.

As a matter of interest, if bacteria start to reproduce in the small intestines, your immune system destroys them, and so they are not tolerated everywhere! This makes sense, as microbes there would be eating our nutrients, and would be in direct competition with you. If bacteria start to colonise your small intestine it is called small intestine bacterial overgrowth (**SIBO**); and your immune system responds to destroy them in that area.

So the supply of soluble fibre as their food explains how our microbiome benefit from living with us, but I said earlier in the book that we have a commensal and also a symbiotic relationship with these bacteria. In other words, as well as tolerating each other we also help each other in some way. So how do we benefit? It turns out that gut microbes are not only protective (both as described above and also by crowding out 'bad' bacteria) but they are also positively beneficial and essential for life! We can read about the benefits of having these commensal bacteria in the next chapter.

Take home message

- You have trillions of bacterial cells living in your colon, and these, together with some other microbes like yeasts, comprise your microbiome.
- The microbes appear to invade your gut prior to you developing an established immune system and appear to play an important role in the development of that immune system, early in infancy.
- Because your gut microbiome coevolved with you, and because your gut bacteria has an epigenetic control over your TLR4 gene, which prevents your immune system from recognising *specific* bacteria as 'foreign', your immune cells do not kill your gut bacteria while they remain within the colon.
- SIBO, which is small intestine bacterial overgrowth, results in those bacteria that have colonised your *small* intestine being destroyed by your immune cells, which shows that microbes are only tolerated in the large intestine, and, more specifically, the colon.

Chapter Six

The Benefits of having Commensal Bacteria in Your Gut

1. Commensal bacteria protect you from gut injury

Ten years ago it was recognised that activation of Toll-like Receptors by commensal bacteria is also critical for protection against gut injury, which may offer an additional explanation of why these bacteria have been tolerated during our co-evolution over thousands of years. However these bacteria are not merely tolerated, as the host-bacterial interaction may be necessary for intestinal balance (homeostasis).

2. Commensal bacteria provide you with an energy source

If our bodies didn't have these commensal microbes, we wouldn't be able to utilize some of the undigested carbohydrates we eat, because some types of gut microbes have enzymes that human cells lack for breaking down certain carbohydrates (polysaccharides). So the microbes benefit us by fermenting undigested carbohydrates and fibre that we are unable to digest; utilising the energy from them. We mentioned this earlier when we said that the microbes use soluble fibre as a food source. What we didn't say earlier was that the result of this is that they create a fuel of short-chain fatty acids, which our body *can* then use.

In fact, without our gut microbes we may have to consume many more calories just to survive! This was discovered in 1983, when mice bred without gut microbes needed 30% more calories than mice with their normal gut microbes.

The most important of the fatty acids (short chain fatty acids, SCFA) which are produced by our gut bacteria and secreted into the gut, for use by us, are:

- **Butyrate**, which the lining of the colon uses for energy,
- **Propionates**, used by the liver; and
- **Acetates**, used by muscle tissue.

The above products are also beneficial in maintaining the barrier in the gut lining.

3. Commensal bacteria are more than useful, they are essential to life

The microbiome is also *essential* to life, as intestinal bacteria also play a role in making products that our body needs. For example:

- **Vitamin B3, B5, B6 and B12, Biotin, and Vitamin K**
- **Folate (for folic acid)**
- **Short Chain Fatty acids (like butyrate)**

In addition to producing these essential vitamins and other products, your gut bacteria also make enzymes which modify substances into a form that your body *can* then use (this is called metabolising them). For example, by producing specific enzymes the bacteria can:

- **Metabolise bile acids**
- **Metabolise sterols** (which occur naturally in plants, animals, and fungi; the most familiar animal sterol being cholesterol)
- **Metabolise xenobiotics** (foreign compounds, including therapeutic drugs, antibiotics and food).

In fact, at least thirty commercially available drugs (also referred to as xenobiotics) are metabolised by bacterial enzymes.

- **They also make analogues (similar in structure) of neurotransmitters that you have in your brain.** One example of this is serotonin, which makes you feel happy. Although these 'neurotransmitters' are not identical to the human ones, they are similar enough for the brain to respond to them as if they were identical. Scientists now estimate that 90% of serotonin is made in the gut.

• **They also aid intestinal cells to produce serotonin.** There are three types of cell that produce serotonin in the gut, and these are immune cells, nerve cells, and enterochromaffin (EC) cells. In a study last year, the EC cells of germ-free mice (those without a gut microbiome) produced around 60% less serotonin than the mice with normal gut bacteria, but when the microbiome of the mice was replaced, their EC cells began producing normal levels of serotonin, showing that the under-production of serotonin can be reversed.

We have so many bacteria in our gut that, as we said, there are ten times more bacterial cells than human cells in the gut, but they also have around a hundred times as many genes (in total) as there are in the human genome.

Not that having more genes is really an indicator of anything, as some plants have more genes than humans too, but it explains why the gut microbiome can metabolize many compounds in ways that humans can't; and that is because they have different enzymes to us (produced by genes that we do not have). Over 40 therapeutic (e.g. prodrugs) and food compounds are known to be modified by the gut microbes, converting inactive products into their useable forms.

4. Commensal Bacteria help us to utilise the drugs we take

For example, the prodrug *Sulfasalazine*, prescribed for **ulcerative colitis**, remains *inactive* until it reaches the colon, where enzymes made by the gut microbiome convert it into its *active* form. Our gut microbes also activate antioxidants and anti-inflammatory components of fruits, vegetables, cereals, and coffee; and at least thirty commercial drugs are metabolised by your gut bacteria. Because of this, the effects of drug treatments can vary enormously between different individuals, and personalising human drug treatments to increase the efficacy of the drugs and also to decrease adverse reactions (a system called pharmacogenomics) is now a very real possibility.

However, environmental factors like a person's nutrition, age, disease, microbiome diversity and interactions between other drugs also affect drug metabolism, their efficiency, and their toxicity; and so it will not be enough to merely look at a person's DNA (a common theme that is developing throughout this book).

In addition to a drug-gene reaction an even *more* personalised drug treatment has been proposed to take into account a variety of factors, including diet, lifestyle, environment, gut microbiome as well as your genes. Tests to determine your responses to potential drugs are relatively easy, and can be done from blood and urine samples. This new personalised approach to drug treatment will make drugs more effective and should hopefully reduce their toxicity.

[*Some additional science for those who are interested in terminology (not necessary unless you are interested!).* **'Pharmaco-genomics'** = *drug and gene interactions.* **'Pharmaco-metabonomics'** = *drug and environmental factors (diet, gut microbiome, lifestyle, environment) and gene interaction. This is also called your metabolic phenotype*]

5. Commensal Bacteria can detoxify foods

In addition, they actively protect us from things like oxalates, found in the food that we eat, which can cause kidney stones and renal failure; and our microbiome makes the enzymes that we need to *detoxify* it. In fact, humans cannot make these enzymes and so these bacteria are essential to our health. The gut microbiome also makes enzymes that *inactivate* some drugs, which we cannot do, and this is an emerging area of research.

6. Commensal Bacteria can protect us from harmful bacteria

As well as all of these active ways that the microbiome is beneficial to us, the microbes also passively protect us, by crowding out our gut so that harmful microbes can't find a space to attach to you.

This crowding out also occurs between different types of commensal bacteria and also between bacteria and other microbes like yeasts; and, as well as crowding out the area, they can also produce anti-microbial chemicals that defend you against harmful invaders.

7. Commensal Bacteria can protect us from chronic disorders

For example, stress can cause abnormal brain plasticity (plasticity means that your brain can alter the function and structure of different parts of itself in some way). It can also reduce the amount of new nerves that the brain produces, which are needed for normal brain development, learning and repair. Stress also impacts many other areas of the body. Commensal bacteria can protect us from this happening by reducing the effects of the stress in the first place. As well as protecting us from stress, the gut microbiome protects us in many other ways, interacting with our immune system, and preventing or reversing the effects of many other triggers of chronic disorders (which may result in long term damage, and even cancer). You can read more about this in the chapter on solutions.

8. Commensal bacteria programme your immune system

Certain commensal bacteria help to develop your immune system, which, in turn, tolerates their presence in your gut. Your gut bacteria communicate with both your innate immune system and also your acquired immune system. Because 'good' bacteria actively shape a healthy immune system, the absence of some of these bacteria can lead to **allergies, chronic disease** and **cancer**. The good news is that, in many cases, this can be prevented or even reversed (see the chapter on solutions).

Take home message

- The 100 trillion microbes that live in your gut are critical to health. The benefits of having commensal bacteria living in your gut are:
- They protect you from gut injury.
- They provide you with an essential energy source.
- They help to maintain the barrier in the gut lining.
- They make essential products like vitamins, folate and short chain fatty acids (like butyrate) from the food that you eat.
- They make enzymes which help you to utilise drugs and bile acids
- They make neurotransmitters like serotonin, the 'happy' hormone
- They can detoxify foods
- They protect you from other bacteria which can be harmful
- They protect you from getting chronic disorders.
- They programme the body's immune system.
- They build and maintain the gut wall, which protects your body from outside invaders.
- By their physical presence, they block harmful microbes from attaching to the gut.
- They produce anti-microbial chemicals that defend you against pathogens.

An impressive list! We can now see why our microbiome is one of the key systems in our body for maintaining our health! I just mentioned that they protect you from other 'harmful' (pathogenic, disease causing) bacteria, and so how do we know which bacteria are good (and live with us commensally) and which ones are pathogenic and need to be kept out at all costs?! I needed to find out what our gut microbiome consisted of, and you can read more about this in the next chapter.

Chapter Seven

What Does Your Gut Microbiome Consist Of?

So far we have seen how the gut microbes become established, why we tolerate them, how they can be protective against damage, enable us to thrive and also help to maintain a healthy balance in the gut. When your gut microbiome is in balance, it can be highly beneficial to digestion, absorption of nutrients, and your immune health.

Essential stuff, so what happens when that balance changes and how/why does it change? What, if any, are the effects on our health? What does out of balance mean exactly? What are these commensal bacterial strains, and why are they different to the ones which cause us harm?

I started with my first question:

Which bacteria should we have in our gut?

Bear with me on this, as there is a lot of information!

Please note: If you prefer not to read about these bacteria at the moment, you can go straight to the take home message in a few pages and continue from there.

There have been two major scientific papers published in recent years on the human gut microbiome which show a huge diversity of bacterial species, but 98% of these species belong to only four families (called phyla):

- Firmicutes (64%),
- Bacteroidetes (23%),
- Proteobacteria (8%), and
- Actinobacteria (3%)

Although these are the estimated percentages from the studies, the current ongoing worldwide study of the human microbiome will, no doubt, reveal a more accurate picture. The human microbiome also contains some viruses, fungi and other microbes.

In this chapter, and in the chapter on solutions, we can see how some of these bacteria are available to take as a probiotic, and how they are useful in treating chronic disorders.

So *Firmicutes* and *Bacteroidetes* are the most dominant bacteria in your gut, but don't be surprised if you haven't heard of them! These names will not be familiar to most of us, but some of the bacterial species that fall *within* these phyla probably *will* be more familiar to you, as we see them in yoghurt drinks for example.

Bacterial species from the phylum *Firmicutes*:

Lactobacillus

These bacteria only have one outer membrane and are more delicate than others, and so can be destroyed more easily by things like antibiotics. This is why it may be useful to replace these bacteria, by taking a probiotic which contains them.

There are many *Lactobacillus* species and are usually written as L plus the name of the species, for example **L. acidophilus**.

Lactobacillus help to ferment vegetable fibre that you cannot digest and one of the end results of this fermentation is that the bacteria produce lactic acid, which increases the acidity in the gut slightly, which, in turn, is harmful to pathogens. Lactic acid can also help humans to digest lactose found in dairy products.

Lactobacillus have many functions, one of which is that they are involved in the conversion of glutamate to gamma-amino butyric acid (GABA) a neurotransmitter which calms down the brain. GABA dysfunction or deficiency is linked to many chronic disorders including **anxiety, behavioural changes such as Attention Deficit Disorder, epilepsy, depression, defects in synapses between nerves** (which could impact on **learning** and **memory**) and **Alzheimer's disease**. Some strains of *Lactobacillus* may be more efficient than others in preventing or reversing disorders and you can read more about this in the chapter on solutions.

The *Lactobacillus* that you may be familiar with include the following:

L. acidophilus –Alleviates sad thoughts and may prevent **depression**. It also makes vitamin K, and maintains the intestinal barrier, which protects us from immune responses to food and prevents bacteria moving out of the intestines. This in turn protects us from gut infections and **irritable bowel disorders**. It is used in some probiotics ('For Every Day Extra Strength', by Optibac, for example).

L. rhamnosus - May be helpful in cases of small intestinal bacterial overgrowth (**SIBO**), **anxiety, depression, Alzheimer's disease** and possibly **epilepsy** and **autism**. It is also used in some probiotics ('For Every Day' by Optibac for example).

L. brevis - It makes the neurotransmitter GABA (gamma-amino butyric acid), which reduces anxiety and depression. It can survive in the gastrointestinal tract in humans and can therefore be used as a probiotic.

L. helveticus – The *L. helviticus* strain R0052, in combination with *Bifidobacterium longum* R0175, reduces anxiety, chronic stress and psychological stress. It is also used as a probiotic.

L. rossiae – one of the strains *proven* to make **vitamin B12** (cobalamin), **vitamin B2** (riboflavin) and **folate**, although many other strains of *Lactobacillus* may also make them, as they share similar genes. It also has genes which can make amino acids, and so may covert glutamate to GABA, which is a calming neurotransmitter, reducing anxiety and depression.

L. kimchi - found in the Korean fermented-vegetable food kimchi.

Some *Lactobacillus* strains also have a tolerance to stress in the gut, can inhibit food borne pathogens and also create immune responses, such as stimulating antibody formation or inhibiting the innate immune (white blood cell) activity (unpublished results).

Although I mentioned that some of the above bacteria are found in **probiotics** (essentially a live supply of 'good' bacteria and yeasts that confer a health benefit on the host, and are naturally found in the microbiome); I also mentioned kimchi, a fermented Korean food. Kimchi is also a *prebiotic*, and prebiotics are a source of food for probiotics to grow, multiply and survive in the gut. Those like kimchi and raw sauerkraut can also be a source of living probiotics. Essentially, prebiotics are plant fibres (soluble fibre) which we can't digest but are a great food source for 'good' bacteria in the gut to increase in number.

- *Good sources of soluble fibre are things like black beans, cannellini beans, butterbeans, lentils, brussel sprouts, oats and chickpeas, as well as many vegetables.*

Bacterial species from the phylum *Bacteroidetes*

The most well studied, and the most dominant in the gut microbiome are *Bacteroides fragilis*.

Bacteroides (and note the difference here between the species, *Bacteroides*, and the very similar name of the family (phylum) *Bacteroidetes* that they belong to) are *less* easily destroyed by antibiotics. They are generally commensal, only causing disease if they move from the gut to other areas of the body (for example during surgery).

Breast-fed infants have very few *Bacteroides* in their faeces until after they are weaned. Until then, most of the gut microbiome, in infants, are *Bifidobacterium*. (Interestingly, a change in the microbiome upon weaning may also be linked to **Type 1 diabetes** but more studies are needed.)

B. fragilis have been identified as a probiotic that is beneficial for GI problems in people with **autism spectrum disorders (ASD)**, although it is unlikely that a probiotic alone could reverse ASD completely as the causes of ASD are complex. However, research into this subject is very sparse so far, and, as diet does play a significant role in many chronic disorders, treatment with prebiotics and probiotics is worth considering. (I discuss ASD later in the book, in the chapter on the gut-brain connection. Yes there is one!).

Bacterial species from the phylum *Proteobacteria*

Proteobacteria are only found in very low abundance in your gut microbiome, but I will mention here that an increase in the abundance of these bacteria has been linked to gallstones.

I mention this only to illustrate that a balanced gut microbiome is necessary for health.

Bacterial species from the phylum *Actinobacteria*

Another lactic acid–producing bacteria that also benefits from prebiotic food is *Bifidobacterium*, a species of the phyla *Actinobacteria*. As with the bacteria described above, it is also found in the microbiome of your colon. Like *Lactobacillus*, it produces lactic acid, and can convert glutamate to gamma-amino butyric acid (GABA), a calming neurotransmitter in the central nervous system that prevents **anxiety** and **depression**.

Bifidobacterium were first discovered in the faeces of breast-fed infants in 1899 by Tissier, who thought that they may protect the infant from diarrhoea. In 1900 he administered live *bifidobacteria* to infants with diarrhoea with successful results (*one of the first times that probiotics were used as a treatment for ill-health*).

Breaking news:

- More recent research has established that human milk contains certain complex carbohydrate/sugars that are not designed to feed the infant, as they are not easily digested and so pass through to the infant's gut, where they can be consumed by gut *bacteria*. In other words, human milk is designed to feed both the infant and the infant's gut microbiome! It is the equivalent of soluble plant fibre.
- More precisely, this 'microbiome food' in the milk is favoured by *B. breve and B. infantis* (see below) and so these bacteria tend to predominate in the baby until it is weaned, after which their gut microbiome becomes more diverse. As these bacteria protect the infant from diarrhoea, they may also protect against other disorders. They are used in probiotics.

B. Infantis – mainly found in human babies prior to weaning. The microbes are thought to be supplied via human milk, which also contains some food which, paradoxically, passes through the baby's digestive tract into the large intestine; where it feeds the gut microbes rather than the infant. This suggests that human milk plays a role in the type of bacteria which will favourably consume this food and so colonise the gut of the baby. In other words, human milk contains a soluble fibre which nurtures a healthy microbiome in the infant prior to weaning. It is used in probiotics for infants (Optibac sell one).

Other bacteria in the infant microbiome can include *B. longum*, *B. breve*, and/or *B. bifidum*. *B. infantis* does not produce gas (as some other bacteria do), which may avoid pain of trapped wind in a small digestive system (my opinion). A meta-analysis showed that *B.*

infantis reduced pain, bloating, and bowel movement difficulty in children with Irritable Bowel Syndrome symptoms. These bacteria can be found in the probiotic 'For Babies and Children' by Optibac.

B. Longum – *B. longum* R0175, in combination with *L. helveticus* R0052 reduces **anxiety, chronic stress** and **psychological stress**. These can be found in some probiotics (Optibac 'For Every Day', for example).

Take Home message

- There are many bacterial strains, and I only mention some of them, but, in summary, they are essential for your health and wellbeing!
- Before I continue, I will just say that I have added information (taken from scientific studies) to the particular strains listed, but they may also have many other functions, other than those listed
- Human breast milk contains food specifically for a baby's gut bacteria.

Although gut bacteria play the most important role in your gut by far, other microbes can also be commensal. One of these is the yeast **Candida Albicans**, which aids digestion, so let us find out a bit more about *Candida* in particular, and yeast in general.

Fungi (yeast)

As we already mentioned, not all bacteria living in your gut are the same, and not all thrive on the same type of foods. Some bacteria thrive on the soluble fibre from plants that we eat (but that we are unable to digest), whereas other microbes can survive on junk food. This also applies to microbes like the yeast *Candida albicans* which can thrive very nicely on sugar; so what you eat, digest and absorb, determines which type of microbes survive in your gut. Some of these microbes contribute towards a healthy body and mind, whereas others contribute towards having chronic disorders.

In healthy individuals, yeast, like *Candida* species, are commensal, and all humans have these yeast (fungi) in their microbiome. There has been very little research on the yeast in our gut until recently, but studies in 2015 suggest that the yeast in the gut can play a role in human health. For example, **Inflammatory Bowel Disease (IBD)** in children was shown to be associated with a reduced diversity of both the yeast and commensal bacteria in the gut, together with an overgrowth of *Candida*. Healthy children do not have this abundance of *Candida albicans* in their gut, and have mostly *Cladosporium* yeast instead.

In fact, although there are far fewer yeast cells than commensal bacteria, their impact on human health is significant, and it appears that the role that yeast plays in the development of inflammatory diseases, as mentioned above, and also in metabolic disorders, like **obesity**, has been underestimated.

However, as with most things, nature favours balance, and *Candida* in the gut, which aids in digestion of food, is self-regulated by expression of its own EFH1 gene, which favours commensalism rather than candidiasis (an acute condition where overabundance of *Candida* can result in infection of the host).

In spite of this self-regulation, the incidence of serious infections with *Candida albicans* in humans is on the rise. The question is why. The use of immunosuppressive drugs like steroids and broad-spectrum **antibiotics** have both been recognized as risk factors (as have some infections like pancreatitis). This would make sense, as killing off pathogenic bacteria with antibiotics also, unfortunately, kills off some of the commensal bacteria in our gut. This leaves a nice space in the gut lining for the yeast to take hold.

Before anyone with **IBD** decides to kill off their *Candida* yeast, this rise in *Candida* infection may not be a problem with the *Candida per se* but could just be indicators of an imbalance between bacterial and fungal commensal microbes living together in the gut, leading to a potential overgrowth of Candida, which would then lead to infection and invasion; which may explain the rise in Candida infections. If this is the case, then returning the gut microbiome and gut yeast population to homeostasis may be the answer. This would involve inoculation of the gut with probiotics to restore the population of commensal bacteria, for example after taking antibiotics, and also supplements to aid in bringing the overgrowth of *Candida* back to normal levels, which can be found in the chapter on supplements later in the book.

Neurotransmitters

I mentioned neurotransmitters above, and that some gut bacteria are associated with them in some way, and so before I continue I will briefly explain what neurotransmitters are.

Neurotransmitters communicate information in our brain and body, by relaying signals between nerve cells (neurons). Your brain uses neurotransmitters to tell your **heart** to beat and your **stomach** to digest food. They can also affect **mood, sleep, concentration** and **weight**, and so the levels of neurotransmitters need to be in balance. However, neurotransmitter levels can be depleted in many ways, for example by **stress,** a poor diet, toxins, drugs (including prescription ones), alcohol and caffeine; so it isn't difficult to see how our lifestyle can impact on our health!

There are two kinds of neurotransmitters, and they are called either **excitatory**, as they stimulate the brain (like **glutamate**), or **inhibitory**, as they calm the brain and help create balance (like **GABA**). Inhibitory neurotransmitters balance mood and can be easily depleted if excitatory neurotransmitters are overactive. One neurotransmitter that many of us are familiar with is **serotonin,** which is a calming neurotransmitter, and so it makes us feel happier as it reduces anxiety. Serotonin also regulates **carbohydrate cravings,** your **sleep cycle, digestion,** and even controls **pain levels.** Low serotonin levels are also associated with a decreased **immune** system function.

Like everything else in your body, neurotransmitters need to be in balance for optimal health! What may surprise you is that your gut microbes can make some of these neurotransmitters, and so by restoring, feeding and keeping a healthy balanced gut **microbiome,** you can also have healthy balanced neurotransmitters! You can read more about this in chapter ten, on the gut-brain connection.

Hormones

I also mentioned hormones, and so I will briefly mention these here too. Hormones are produced by endocrine glands (like the thyroid gland) and are sent to different parts of the body to exert their effect. For example, thyroid hormones affect *every single cell in your body* and have several major functions. They:

- Control metabolism, resulting in weight loss or weight gain.
- Slow down or speed up the heartbeat (can cause feelings of anxiety)
- Raise or lower body temperature.
- Affect the speed that food moves through the digestive tract.
- Control the way muscles contract.
- Control how quickly dying cells are replaced.

You can see why it is important to have balanced hormone levels! However, don't be too worried about this, as following the solutions suggested later in the book should keep your hormones in balance without you having to think about it.

Take home message

- Your gut microbiome is diverse, and consists of different strains of bacteria, together with some other microbes, like fungi.
- Some gut bacteria are more easily destroyed than others (for example by antibiotics)
- When our gut microbiome becomes out of balance, it can lead to chronic disease
- Neurotransmitters and hormones need to be in balance for physical and mental health; but taking the steps in the chapter on solutions should do this without you having to give it a second thought. However, if you have taken all the steps and still have a problem, it is best to have your hormone levels checked.

Chapter Eight

Your Gut Microbiome and Chronic Disorders

Why is the microbiome a key system for long term health?

There is growing evidence that dysbiosis (imbalance) of the gut microbiome is associated with the development of many chronic disorders, including **inflammatory bowel disease, irritable bowel syndrome (IBS), coeliac disease, allergy, asthma, metabolic syndrome, cardiovascular disease, diabetes, thyroid disorders, rheumatoid arthritis** and **obesity,** to name but a few; and we read how our gut microbiome can become out of balance by eating a diet poor in fruit and vegetables and also by taking antibiotics. But what if our gut microbiome was never in balance in the first place? In other words, what if the gut microbiome that we are born with makes us susceptible to some chronic disorders?

The gut microbiome that you are born with

This has been investigated over recent years and, although we know that we are inoculated with our microbiome while in the womb and during the first months of life, recent research suggests that some of the genes in our DNA can influence which bacteria are *able* to colonise our gut, and these are the genes in our body which control immunity. In other words, the genes that allow us to detect which is 'self' and which is 'foreign'.

Each of us has a unique set of genes, particularly those that allow each person's immune system to react to a wide range of foreign invaders. Although many of these versions of the immune genes are very similar to one another, it is these slight differences which *may* determine whether a particular strain of commensal bacteria is seen as safe or not, and so our unique set of HLA genes will determine, to a degree, which gut bacteria we have. **But do not be alarmed!** Always remember that having specific genes which make you *susceptible* to a particular disorder does NOT mean that you will get the disorder; and much depends on your diet and lifestyle. More importantly, in spite of our genes, it *is* possible to change your microbiome and restore health, and you can read more about this in the chapter on solutions.

We also read, in chapter two, 'Your genes and your DNA', that your diet affects the genes of your children and grandchildren, by 'marking' their genes with information about the availability of food. In addition to this 'epigenetic marking' our children also inherit our microbiome, which may be beneficial to the environment they are being born into, or not. For example, the bacteria family *Firmicutes* may encourage more fat storage than *Bacteroidetes*, which may be beneficial in times of food scarcity; but most western diets are not short of food, so if we have an abundance of *Firmicutes* bacteria compared to *Bacteroidetes* we may become **overweight**, and **obese**, which can then lead to ill health. The story is more complicated than that, but you see how some bacteria labelled as 'bad' can actually be 'good' in different circumstances; in this case depending on the scarcity or abundance of a food supply.

But do not despair! For those reading this and feeling despondent, in case they are trying to lose weight and fear that they have too many *Firmicutes*, fear not. Bacteria have a short lifespan and so they are being replaced regularly. But they have taken a place in our gut and crowded out other bacteria haven't they? That is true, but things like probiotics (capsules containing live bacteria), prebiotics (certain foods that optimally feed our microbiome) and a change of certain foods that we eat, have been shown to change our microbiome, in only a few days. In extreme cases, a microbiome can be transplanted from a 'healthy' person into one suffering from a chronic disorder, and I will talk more about this later in this chapter and also in the chapter on solutions (it is called **faecal transplant**), but let me tell you now that it works!!

So we know that our immune genes may determine which bacteria we have living in our gut, and that we inherit our microbiome, and also that food can exert an epigenetic control over our DNA; BUT, we also know that, although some gut microbiomes are associated with chronic disorders, this can be addressed by changing and avoiding some foods and restoring our gut microbiome in most cases. Even **autoimmune** disorders may be reversed if they are treated before the immune system destroys a particular organ; and examples of a chronic disorder being reversed can be seen in **coeliac disease** (by removing the trigger of gluten from the diet) and **type 2 diabetes** (by making diet and lifestyle changes).

The gut microbiome that you have today

Whatever microbiome we are born with, the ratio of *Firmicutes* to *Bacteroidetes* evolves during different life stages, although diet, and possibly probiotics, should maintain a healthy gut microbe balance throughout life.

The change in numbers of *Bifidobacterium* in our gut microbiome is also thought to decline with age, as well as in response to diet. However, regular consumption of fermented foods, and/or use of a probiotic supplement, should maintain a healthy microbiome.

We know that antibiotics kill some of the bacteria in your gut, especially more 'fragile' ones like *Lactobacillus*, and so your gut microbiome needs to be restored if you have ever taken antibiotics.

Diet and environmental conditions can influence the different species of bacteria in our gut microbiome even from birth For example, a breast-fed, full-term infant has mainly *bifidobacteria* in their microbiome, whereas formula-fed infants have mainly *coliforms*.

However, please remember that it is also possible to change your, and your infant's, gut microbiome by taking probiotics and eating a prebiotic diet, so there is no need to be alarmed by the differences in the microbiome of different babies if you had a baby by **C-section** or are not **breastfeeding**. If any children do seem to have gut problems, there are even specific probiotics available for paediatric gastrointestinal conditions.

- *Whatever gut microbiome you were born with, or have now, you can change it for a healthy balanced microbiome; and there is more about this in the chapter on solutions.*

Eating for a healthy microbiome

There are hundreds of studies to show that the health of your body and mind is linked to what you eat, digest and absorb (I mention absorb because it doesn't matter what you eat if your body doesn't absorb it!).

One meta-analysis showed that eating a high daily intake of fruit and vegetables reduces the risk of several chronic diseases, including **hypertension, coronary heart disease, strokes, cancer, prevention of weight gain, type 2 diabetes, certain eye diseases, dementia, osteoporosis, asthma, chronic obstructive pulmonary disorder,** and **rheumatoid arthritis**; as well as promoting health.

Your diet is one of the easiest things to modify in terms of lifestyle changes, but can it make that much difference to your health? The answer to that seems to be yes, and it can be seen in studies where adult human faecal microbes were transplanted into germ-free mice (those with no microbiome at all). In these studies, the same human diversity of bacterial colonisation stabilised in the gut of the mice; and this was inherited by future generations. It is a procedure called **faecal transplantation** and you can read more about this in the chapter on solutions, as it is being used to treat some human diseases.

So far so good but where does diet come into this? Well, it was found that if the diet of the mice was changed from a low-fat, plant rich diet to a high-fat, high-sugar 'western' diet, the microbiome changed *within a single day*. In addition to a change in bacterial diversity, there was also, as a consequence, a change in the bacterial products being made; which resulted in the 'humanised' mice gaining fat.

This could be *reversed* if the mice received another transplant of a healthy human gut microbiome; but, although this colonisation of a healthy balanced microbiome affected the structure of the microbiome community in the mice initially, the beneficial effects could always be rapidly altered by diet.

So, to summarise, eating a variety of vegetables, and a reasonable amount of them (half of your dinner plate), together with a little fruit, will feed your 'good' bacteria with the soluble fibre they need to survive and thrive; and these 'good' bacteria will make products that are beneficial to your health. Not only do those bacterial products contribute towards a healthy body, we read in the chapter on the benefits of having commensal bacteria, that some 'good' bacteria also produce neurotransmitters which make us feel happier, and so they also contribute towards a healthy mind. You can read more about all of this in the chapter on solutions.

However, sometimes life feels like a struggle, and we can feel overwhelmed by cravings for foods/drinks which we know are not good for us, so can we do anything about that? Yes we can!

As some of us struggle with **cravings** for sugar, is there anything we can eat which can help reduce those cravings? We know that an overload of *Candida albicans* can make us crave processed sugar, and so restoring the levels of good microbes in our gut will help; but sugar and quickly digested carbohydrates like potatoes and pasta causes a surge of your insulin levels, which can then cause sugar cravings (and can also be linked to obesity and Type II diabetes, both 'lifestyle' diseases); so are there any solutions for this to be found in your diet? Well there may be, and the answer may lie in beans and something called '**The Second Meal Effect**'.

The '**second meal effect**' means that eating legumes, like beans, reduces the speed at which the glucose from the food that you eat is digested and absorbed, and may also reduce the actual calories absorbed. This applies to food eaten at the same meal, the following meal, or even the following day. In other words, it makes the food that you eat be absorbed less quickly by your body, and can even reduce the calories absorbed from your meal.

You will no longer experience the insulin rush created if you ate a meal with only sugars and easily digested carbohydrates like pasta and potatoes, with a corresponding craving to eat sugary foods as your blood sugar levels temporarily drop (the craving for 'something sweet' after a carbohydrate laden dinner).

This is great for all of us, but could be particularly useful for diabetics who have to take insulin, as it could reduce the amount of insulin they need, but why is this important?

First of all let me explain the difference between **Type I** and **Type 2 diabetes**. **Type I diabetes** is an autoimmune disease, occurring early in life. It results in destruction of the pancreas cells, which make insulin, and so patients need to take insulin all of their life; whereas **Type II diabetes** is a disorder brought on later in life by diet and lifestyle, and it can be reversed.

Although I said that **Type I diabetes** can't be reversed, which it can't, it is possible to reduce the *amount* of insulin a **Type I diabetic** needs. People in the diabetic community have focused on blood sugar, and getting it into 'normal' ranges, so that a Type I diabetic can eat what they want and then adjust their blood sugar with medication; **insulin**. However, a reduction in the *amount* of insulin needed also reduces the risk of other chronic disorders, and for a Type I diabetic, this means they can extend their life and have a better health, without the highs and lows.

[I should say here that although diabetes involves high blood sugar, it is not purely a disorder of high blood sugar, which is called hyperglycaemia. Diabetes is much more complicated, and is a complex metabolic condition].

- A study into the benefits, or otherwise, of a high carbohydrate diet indicated that only the soluble fibre found in legumes, vegetables, and fruits improved blood glucose levels and cholesterol metabolism, and that eating only fibre supplements did not work. The fibre has to come with the whole food for it to be effective.

Soluble fibre, particularly that found in beans, oats, Brussel sprouts and flax seeds, also reduces **LDL,** the 'bad' cholesterol that is linked to **coronary heart disease.**

Eating fruits and vegetables have also been shown to protect against **cardiovascular disease** and **anxiety,** and also improve **brain function**; because, by feeding the gut microbes, they in turn protect us from chronic disorders.

Breaking news!

- Finally, exciting new research involving hundreds of people, published in November 2015, has proven that eating for your microbiome can change the microbes in your gut, and that this can reduce your chances of getting chronic disorders. The research showed that we do not all respond in the same way to the same food. For example, some people had raised blood glucose after eating bananas, while others did not; and this was linked to the different bacteria that they had in their gut. After a few days of making a change in their diet, the researchers found that the gut microbiome of the people in the study also changed! Exciting stuff! All of the research I have read also shows this, but to have one piece of recent and ongoing research that supports all of my findings; while specifically looking at people eating in their normal way, eating what they normally eat, looking at the times of day that they eat, their lifestyle and their environment, is very exciting.

Restoring your gut bacteria with probiotics

As some of your 'good' bacteria may have been killed off by antibiotics, diet and lifestyle, this suggests that they need to be replaced, and this is now possible by taking a broad based probiotic. Why do I say broad based? Well research shows that the more diverse a microbiome is, the more chance there is for it to remain in balance. The more diversity there is, the less chance there is of large numbers of one specific bacteria dying off and being replaced by a large group of another specific bacteria. It is much less likely to see a dominance of one strain in other words, which leads to an imbalance. You can find much more about which probiotics to take in the chapter on solutions.

Take home message

- Eating vegetables, and maybe beans and other legumes, can feed your good gut bacteria and contribute to your health; however, we read earlier that some 'good' bacteria are fragile, and can be destroyed, for example by antibiotics; and so restoring your good bacteria, by re-inoculating your gut, may also be needed. These live bacteria are called **probiotics**, and they can be found in either probiotic capsules, or in fermented foods like Kimchi and raw sauerkraut. I say raw because heat would kill off the beneficial microbes. Look for fermented vegetables that use salt, rather than vinegar, or make your own!

- Your gut bacteria can be restored with live bacteria, and these are called probiotics. The specific probiotics for different disorders can be found in the chapter on solutions.

So, in an ideal world, after restoring and feeding our gut microbiome, and finding which probiotics to take, we now have a healthy restored microbiome that, in turn, will keep us healthy and protect us from chronic disorders right? Well the answer is YES, but *only* if we don't damage our intestines with certain drugs, food or other factors, which we can read more about in the next chapter; because this will lead to inflammation of the intestines. This, in turn, weakens the attachment of the good bacteria and they get flushed out of our body; which leads to an imbalance in our gut microbiome and we have to start all over again!

In addition to causing inflammation inside our intestines, some things actually cause the small intestines (but not the colon) to become leaky. This 'leaky gut', together with an imbalanced gut microbiome, can result in chronic and autoimmune disorders, which we can also read about in the next chapter.

So, we need to know how to protect ourselves from damaging our intestines and getting leaky gut!

Chapter Nine

Damage to the Intestinal Lining, Leaky Gut, Autoimmune and Chronic Disorders

So what can damage your intestines? They can be summarised into three main things, and they are all connected:

1. Drugs – like NSAIDs (they can damage the mucous layer)
2. Infection of the intestines – by bacteria; by cholera (rare)
3. Food – like gluten and dairy

Before I explain these in more detail, I will give a brief summary:

Drugs

The NSAID drugs are taken to relieve chronic pain, but if they are damaging the lining of your intestines you could be on a hamster wheel of 'damage – repair – restore – repeat'. Perhaps you could discuss alternative pain relief with your doctor if you decide to try and cure the root cause of your chronic pain.

Infections

Although most of your gut bacteria live in your colon, some try and make a home in your small intestines, but your body will not tolerate them there. The disorder is called **SIBO** (small intestine bacterial overgrowth).

If you have **SIBO**, a protein in your intestines signals to open up the Tight Junctions to let your (large) immune cells in the blood come into your small intestine and kill the invading bacteria. Once the bacteria have been destroyed and flushed out of your body, (with water that also comes in through the Tight Junctions), the lining of your intestines regains its normal barrier function. The whole thing has corresponding diarrhoea as the bugs are flushed out of the body.

Your body's response to **Cholera** is similar to you having **SIBO**, but instead of the protein in your intestines signally to open the Tight Junctions, it is a toxin in the **cholera** that actually signals to open them; resulting in chronic diarrhoea.

In fact, it was during the research into a vaccine for cholera, which can be life threatening, that the Tight Junctions, and the method of opening them, was discovered, and this led to breaking new information about intestinal permeability; which we refer to, for ease, as **Leaky gut**. This, in turn, led to the understanding of the root cause of chronic and autoimmune disorders. It also led to the understanding of the prevention and even reversal (unless the damage to particular organs was too great) of these autoimmune and chronic disorders. (As a reminder, chronic disorders are disorders that last longer than three months, but do not involve your body attacking its own organs; whereas autoimmune disorders, although also being chronic disorders, also involve your immune cells attacking 'you').

It was this understanding, that your intestines could become 'leaky', because of external triggers (like cholera), that led to the discovery that some foods, like gluten (in wheat, barley and rye) can also open up your Tight Junctions. It also led to the discovery of zonulin, which is the protein in the intestines that opens the Tight Junctions if you have **SIBO**.

Food

The reason why this 'leakiness' led to an understanding of chronic and autoimmune disease is because, for the first time, it was realised that large food particles (from partly digested food) could enter the bloodstream below, and come into contact with immune cells; which, in turn, would recognise the food proteins as 'foreign' and so start to attack them.

However, if the *food* proteins are similar to *human* proteins (like, for example, the thyroid gland), then those antibodies will start to attack 'you'; to be specific, in this example, they will attack your thyroid gland.

This was not thought to be possible until recently, as all immune cells which recognise 'you' were thought to be destroyed before they could enter the bloodstream. However, recent research has established that your T cells that recognise 'self', are *not* destroyed, but are normally not active. It seems possible (my opinion), that these 'self-selecting' T cells could be triggered by these novel (food) proteins, that your immune cells have never come into contact with before (wheat protein doesn't invade your bloodstream normally!); and, although they are not normally activated, this new 'invader' may be such a strong trigger that it is enough to activate those specific T cells. The reason why the damage is organ specific would be because the T cells with 'glycan' recognition patterns for a food (like gluten), will only 'match' the proteins of that one, specific, (similar) human organ (like the thyroid gland for example).

Until more research is done in that area, the current thinking is that, because the food proteins are 'similar' to those of specific organs in your body (like the thyroid gland), then your *active* immune cells get it slightly wrong and start to attack that (human) organ, because of 'molecular mimicry'(explained later in this chapter).

OK, I have explained the process in principle, but you need to see the research right?! (I will not be discussing NSAIDs further). The research into infections/foods causing Leaky gut, and associated chronic/autoimmune disorders, started on different journeys, but met up about sixteen years ago.

In fact, the initial realisation that a food could trigger a chronic disease started way back in the 1940s and so that is where I am going to start. The food was **wheat**, and the disease was **coeliac disease**.

How the link between food and a chronic disorder was made.

The Timeline

- **1940s**

The possibility that a food could be implicated in chronic disorders is not a recent finding, as the link between gluten and **coeliac disease** actually started in the 1940s. During World War II, a paediatric gastroenterologist from the Netherlands, Dr Dicke, observed that deaths from **coeliac disease** (it used to be fatal) dropped from 35% to zero during World War II; but when the war was over, the death rate went back to the pre-war era.

He realised that no wheat had been available during the war, and so, using an elimination diet (removing specific things from the diet, like wheat for example) to determine the trigger of the coeliac disease in infants, he tried them on a diet where only grains containing gluten were eliminated, and everything else in their diet stayed the same. The results proved that gluten was indeed the trigger for **coeliac disease**, and it is how the link between a food (in this case wheat) and a chronic disorder (in this case coeliac disease) was first discovered. It wasn't known exactly how this worked though.

At the time, this research (the link between food and chronic disease) was not pursued by other research teams, because coeliac disease was very rare; and generally, diet was not considered to be a possible trigger for chronic disease (it was not thought that food to could be a trigger because it had to leave the intestines and come into contact with immune cells and it was simply too big to do that).

This area of research was not pursued for decades, but something happened to trigger interest in it again, and that was the increase in the number of people with symptoms of **coeliac disease**; although research was hampered by the fact that accurate diagnostic tests for the disease were limited; until the 1990s.

- **1990**

In the early 1990s, tests (ELISA, enzyme-linked immunosorbent assay tests) for *specific* antibodies (for example those raised against gluten) with an accuracy of 95 per cent became available, but they were costly and difficult to interpret.

- **1997**

In 1997 a test that was specific for **coeliac disease** was determined. Many research teams were now researching causes of other chronic disorders.

- **2000**

Coeliac disease is still a rare disorder today, as we need the genes to make us susceptible to it before we actually get **coeliac disease**, and the numbers of us with those genes are relatively few in number. However, in a study of 3000 adults, studied since the 1970s, to establish the prevalence of **coeliac disease** in the general population in the USA; they found that *the incidence of coeliac disease almost doubled every fifteen years or so.*

1970s	1:500
Mid 1980s	1:250
2000	1:133

From our knowledge, that genes cannot evolve that quickly throughout whole populations at once, this implied that something other than our genes was causing this increase. However, the research also threw up an anomaly. Although all of the people in the study had the (immune) genes that made them susceptible to coeliac disease (the HLA-DQ2 or -DQ8 genes) they didn't all get it at (roughly) the same age. In fact, some people were in their seventies when the disease apparently started. I will explain why this might happen later in the chapter.

At the same time as the study of **coeliac disease** incidence, Dr Fasano and his team were researching a vaccine for the **cholera** bacteria (whose toxin, called *Zot* increases the permeability of the gut lining, causing severe diarrhoea). Although they didn't manage to find a vaccine, in 2000, they discovered a human analogue to *Zot*; a protein they called **zonulin**. (In other words, zonulin was similar to *Zot*). They found that this protein (zonulin), produced by the cells in your intestine, regulated the opening of the Tight Junctions of the lining of the small intestines. What is more, they found that levels of zonulin were raised during the acute phase of **coeliac disease**; as Tight Junctions opened and intestinal permeability (leaky gut) increased.

[We mentioned commensal bacterial overgrowth of the small intestines (SIBO), and infection by pathogenic bacteria (for example cholera), earlier in the book; and that they all trigger an opening of the Tight Junctions, to allow large immune cells to come into the intestines, from the blood supply below, and kill the invading bacteria. However, the difference between most bacterial infections and cholera was that Zot could actually trigger our body to open our Tight Junctions. In other words, because it is similar to our own protein, zonulin, our body responds in the same way; with associated localised inflammation from the immune response].

Infections of the small intestine were also being implicated in other **autoimmune**, **allergic**, and **inflammatory diseases**, by causing this impairment (leaking) of the intestinal barrier.

- **2007**

Discovery that 'junk' DNA (dark matter) controls our genes; and is activated by our diet, our environment and our lifestyle (see the chapter on DNA).

- **2008**

The discovery was made that gluten can also cause chronic *inflammation* of the small intestine (which would disrupt the gut microbiome). In addition, over the last ten years, there has been increasing recognition of an association between disrupted intestinal barrier function and the development of autoimmune and inflammatory diseases. Many other chronic disorders are now coming under the umbrella of autoimmunity in terms of how they should be treated, as they all have a root of chronic inflammation (i.e. caused by a trigger(s) that continually provoke an immune response), and intestinal permeability.

- **2011**

Further research had established that, although there are several triggers of zonulin release, exposure to bacteria and gluten in the intestines are the two most powerful triggers.

We have already mentioned bacterial infection of the small intestines triggering zonulin (SIBO and cholera for example) but why would gluten be a trigger? Haven't we been eating bread for hundreds of years? Well yes we have, but the problem we have with gluten is that we don't digest it that well; and only recent discoveries of accurate testing have given us the ability to make an accurate diagnosis.

Gluten contains a large number of two particular amino acids, called **proline (O)** and **glutamine (O)**; and we don't have the enzymes to break **proline** apart from other amino acids in a protein chain; so instead of breaking the gluten protein into single amino acids we are left with small chains (peptides) of amino acids (we call these peptides 'prolamines').

O-O-O-O-O

One of these peptides is called **gliadin**, and it is this peptide that causes **coeliac disease** in people who have the genes that make them susceptible to it. Other peptides in gluten cause **intestinal inflammation**, and may be linked to **gluten 'sensitivity'**; where you don't have the destruction of intestinal cells found in coeliac disease but still get many of the symptoms of it. You can read more about this later in the chapter.

How Gliadin causes coeliac disease

If these gluten peptides stayed inside the intestines they would just pass out of our body in faeces; but the peptides actually manage to get *out* of our intestines and *into* the bloodstream below (even though, in theory, they shouldn't be able to because they are too big) because gliadin activates the zonulin pathway. In other words:

- Gliadin triggers zonulin which, in turn, opens the Tight Junctions in the intestine, you get **Leaky Gut**, the gliadin passes into your bloodstream and comes into contact with your immune cells. This triggers an immune response against gliadin.

Remember that I just mentioned prolamine peptides (like gliadin), which are made of small chains of proline and glutamine? Well there is an enzyme, found in many areas of our body which binds with proteins which contain these amino acids; and it is called transglutaminase (TG2). One area that this enzyme is found is in the epithelial cells of the small intestine, and it is normally inactive. However, when it comes into contact with gliadin (which it mistakes for one of the proteins that it should bind to) it binds to it and modifies it (changes it a little); to a form that is then recognised by parts of our body (because of the 'lock and key' way that proteins work); and this active form of gliadin is immune-toxic to our body.

In addition to this, because the TG2 has bound to the gliadin, when this combination comes into contact with our immune cells, people with the *gene susceptibility* for **coeliac disease** raise antibodies (also called immunoglobulins - Ig) against the combination.

> • In other words, our body raises antibodies, which will attack both the gliadin *and* the TG2 enzyme. Even without symptoms, 98 percent of people with **coeliac disease** will test positive for TG2-IgA antibodies in their blood while eating gluten. As transglutaminase is found all over the body, this can make coeliac disease a very complicated disorder, impacting on all areas of the body. If you don't have those genes, you may get a chronic disorder, with some symptoms of **coeliac disease**, but you will not raise antibodies against your *own* body tissues and so will not get coeliac disease.

Some people that are genetically susceptible to coeliac disease have a close link to specific HLA genes; but this is not always found in chronic disorders, and even in coeliac disease there is not a 100 per cent association.

> • In fact, **less than 10 percent of people with increased genetic susceptibility progress to clinical disease, suggesting a strong environmental trigger in the pre-disease state. (This may explain why the ladies in the coeliac disease study** (see year 2000 timeline) **did not get the disease until they were in their seventies).**

The gliadin peptide is similar to the cells of the intestinal lining, and so the antibodies raised against gliadin also attack the intestine lining, resulting in the villi, and microvilli, being flattened, affecting the person's ability to digest food. It is an example of molecular mimicry, which isn't normally a problem as food that hasn't been broken down, as we said before, doesn't normally come out of the intestines, and so the immune cells don't normally come into contact with it. It is a condition that is brought about purely because of a system failure in the intestines, and that system failure is triggered by a simple food; gluten.

Another feature of gliadin, and other gluten peptides, is that it stimulates innate immune cells to start an *inflammation* process, and also stimulates cytokine release. As we already read, in the chapter on the immune system, cytokines are messengers, signalling other immune cells to come to the area, starting a cascade of inflammation (they are also involved in the regulation of inflammation, stopping it via a feedback system); and in all chronic inflammation we see a cytokine storm. If the trigger keeps coming (if gluten is eaten) then chronic inflammation (in this case in the intestines) will occur. All because of a simple food.

However, just as the trigger of gluten can start coeliac disease, once the trigger (gluten) is removed from the diet, zonulin levels decrease, the intestine's barrier function returns, auto-antibodies stop being produced, the autoimmune process shuts off, and consequently, the intestinal damage (which is the biological outcome of the autoimmune process) heals completely in coeliac disease. Great news! BUT! If gluten is eaten *at all* the symptoms will return, and so people have to be *very* careful to maintain a gluten-free diet. (Meaning, as we already mentioned, the gluten from wheat, barley and rye). This includes many sauces and ready meals, which can use wheat as a thickener.

- **2012**

Chronic disorders range from **obesity** and **diabetes** to **Alzheimer's disease, thyroid disorders, multiple sclerosis, rheumatoid arthritis** and **depression**, among others; and current thinking is that autoimmunity may not be a disease, but a disorder on a continuum; where your body can become worse over time, with chronic disorder(s), until it develops a full blown autoimmune response. If this is the case, finding the triggers, and preventing these autoimmune responses, is even more critical.

In most cases, increased permeability of the small intestines (leaky gut) precedes disease, including **type I diabetes**, and this can persist at a low level. It may be that other triggers, such as other foods, together with non-food triggers, may cross react and/or place a burden on the body which manifests in low level intestinal inflammation with low level **intestinal permeability** (my opinion). However, by using an elimination diet (see later in this book) and eating whole foods, we should be able to find the triggers of our health problems.

I mentioned earlier (see 'timeline', year 2000), that some people in the study of coeliac incidence in the USA, by Dr Fasano and his team, did not develop **coeliac disease** until later in life, with some in their seventies. If, as it seems, we need to reach a critical burden of a trigger, or triggers, before a full blown autoimmune response occurs; and, as we all have a unique set of immune (HLA) genes, this may also explain why some of us seem to tolerate triggers more than others (my opinion).

'Leaky gut', has now been studied extensively, both for **coeliac disease** and also in relation to other chronic and autoimmune disorders; and it has been found that even disorders *outside* of the gut, like **asthma**, have increased intestinal permeability.

Even disorders characterised as 'brain' disorders, like **multiple sclerosis**, are now known to have an increase in permeability, but this time it is in the blood-brain barrier (BBB), (I call this 'leaky brain'); although they can also have leaky gut. Increased permeability of the BBB was previously thought to be impossible, for similar reasons to those of the gut, in that the barrier is needed to protect the brain. However, Zonulin is found in many epithelial areas of the body, and expression of zonulin also correlates with the degradation of the blood-brain barrier in some brain tumours of glial cells in the brain. As **Alzheimer's disease** also has an association with glial cells it is possible that 'leaky brain' may precede the disease.

Take home message

- A gut microbiome that is out of balance, either because you were born with that or because you have taken antibiotics in your life, or not eaten enough soluble fibre in vegetables in fruits; together with food triggers which cause inflammation inside your intestines, all contribute to the development of chronic disorders, and autoimmune diseases such as type 1 diabetes.
- In addition to what is happening inside your colon, where your microbiome lives, and also inflammation in your small intestines, your small intestines can also become *leaky*; either because you have a bacterial infection there, or because one or more foods trigger your zonulin pathway, leading to an immune response to food, with associated inflammation and possible destruction of your own body tissues (if you have the genes which make you susceptible to specific autoimmune disorders)
- Alterations in the composition of your microbiome can also occur after exposure to various other environmental factors, for example environmental toxins and even prescription drugs.
- **The good news is that these can all be resolved, by eating more vegetables, restoring your gut microbiome (with probiotics) and avoiding food-triggers of inflammation and tissue destruction.** You can read how to

find your own triggers in the chapter on the elimination diet and also the chapter on solutions.

• Many other chronic disorders are now coming under the umbrella of autoimmunity in terms of how they should be treated, as they all have a root of chronic inflammation (i.e. caused by a trigger(s) that continually provokes an immune response), and these chronic disorders range from **obesity** and **diabetes** to **Alzheimer's disease, thyroid disorders, multiple sclerosis, rheumatoid arthritis** and **depression**, among others.

• Current thinking is that autoimmunity may not be a disease, but a disorder on a continuum, where your body can become worse over time until it develops a full blown autoimmune response, developing antibodies against a particular organ in your body. If this is the case, finding the triggers, and preventing these autoimmune responses, is even more critical.

Molecular mimicry

This is when some foreign proteins (in the food and drink we consume) are very similar in structure to parts of *human* proteins, and both gluten and the milk from cows are examples of this. Many health problems and autoimmune disorders have now become associated with some of the most commonly consumed foods in the world, such as wheat and milk, because of this molecular mimicry, and that includes both immune and brain disorders. (Normally of course, gluten and milk proteins from dairy products, would never be found in a human bloodstream. They are not pathogenic bacteria or viruses and would not have any way to get into your bloodstream (normally) as they are too big to pass out of your gut). A new study looking at the prevalence of antibodies against wheat and milk proteins in the blood of 400 screened blood donors, found that approximately half of those who reacted to wheat also reacted to brain-based proteins, and the same was found in the subgroup reacting to dairy. This process is called cross-reactivity and it happens because of similarities, molecular mimicry. In other words, if you produce antibodies against dairy, you may also react to gluten; and the target of both of these antibodies can be similar to proteins in the brain, resulting in brain disorders like **multiple sclerosis**.

Now we can see a possible link between our DNA, our digestive system, our gut microbes, our immune system, some foods and many chronic disorders. We just read about Leaky Gut, and that particles that are much larger than amino acids (so peptides or whole proteins) can pass out of your gut into the bloodstream below the gut epithelium. We also just read that these proteins can be very similar in structure to the host proteins (for example the thyroid gland or gut lining). Although the proteins in the food are obviously not *exactly* the same as the human cells, and are different enough to cause an immune response against them, they are *similar* enough for the resulting antibodies (the immunoglobulins like IgE, IgA etc.) that have been made to attack the food protein, to also mistakenly attack the host tissue.

In other words, this is an example of molecular mimicry, where antibodies are made against dairy proteins found in the bloodstream but which then also attack the host thyroid gland cells too, which appear to be similar to the dairy proteins, thereby destroying the thyroid organ. This is why antibodies raised against gliadin (one of the peptides in the protein gluten) also destroy the gut villi, (which flattens these tiny projections, making it difficult to absorb nutrients from the food eaten).

Take home message

- There are Tight Junctions in the small intestine, and if these open when they should not open, this causes intestinal permeability (Leaky Gut).

- The cholera toxin *Zot* can open up these Tight Junctions, as can the human analogue of *Zot,* an intestinal protein called zonulin.
- Zonulin (normally) only opens Tight Junctions if the *small* intestine is colonised by bacteria (SIBO).
- Some proteins, found in viruses, bacteria and some foods, have a similar molecular structure to human proteins. This is called molecular mimicry.

What do we know so far?

1. We know that eating gluten is linked to coeliac disease (an autoimmune disease), and
2. To have an autoimmune disorder the food (in this case gluten) in your gut needs to escape into your bloodstream and come into contact with your immune cells.
3. We also know that the only way this can happen is if you have a leaky gut.
4. Gluten activates zonulin, which leads to Leaky Gut.

Other Possible Causes of Leaky Gut

This is a really simple summary based on many research papers:

Your diet: We have got used to seeing 'foods' on our shelves that include refined sugars and flours, additives, preservatives and flavours, which your body doesn't recognise as food (in its natural state) and this response to the 'foods' can cause inflammation in the gut, which disrupts the mucous lining and microbiome, and so may contribute towards leaky gut.

Chronic Stress: Because stress is actually our 'fight or flight' response, when you are stressed your body puts all of its energy into increasing blood glucose so that you have the extra energy to fight or run; while damping down other things in your body like digestion and your immune system. The problem with an immune system that isn't up to its normal capacity is that it can become overwhelmed by pathogens, which can result in inflammation, for example in the gut. In addition, a dampened down digestive system leads to partially digested food into the small intestine, possible *Candida* yeast overgrowth, bacteria overgrowth in the small intestines (SIBO), infection, parasites and environmental toxins; all conditions which contribute towards leaky gut.

Medication: Some prescription drugs, particularly those given to reduce inflammation, like ibuprofen and diclofenac (NSAIDs) can actually cause inflammation in the gut which may promote an increase in permeability.

Candida overgrowth: *Candida* is found normally in your gut, and is needed in small amounts, but an overgrowth can cause inflammation in the gut and so promote leaky gut.

Zinc deficiency: is needed to maintain a healthy intestinal mucous lining, and so a deficiency may cause leaky gut. Zinc is also needed to aid absorption of vitamin C.

But that still doesn't answer the question as to why we are seeing an *increase* of coeliac disease. I could see how Leaky Gut may explain how the immune cells in our blood system come into contact with otherwise harmless products, like partly digested animal proteins for example, and so recognise them as harmful in the first place, and also how this may lead to autoimmunity in some cases after a response by your acquired immune cells, but what was causing the gut to become more permeable in the first place? The system has evolved over thousands of years not to be leaky, so what was causing this rapid rise in chronic disorders, like **obesity** and **type 2 diabetes**, all related to **Leaky Gut**?

One explanation could be that our food has changed. For example, the dwarf wheat of today has *more* gluten in it than older wheat varieties, so could this explain the increase in coeliac disease?

Certainly from records of American forces personnel taken during the war, coeliac disease existed then, and the prevalence of coeliac disease in the United States has increased dramatically over the last fifty years.

Could the fact that gluten is used extensively in processed food products, bombarding our bodies with gluten be a factor? It is a possibility, as gluten is used as a thickener in many processed foods. The fact that the new processed 'foods', combining ingredients, that are not normally found together, may also confuse our digestive system, but that is only a theory.

- **2013**

The discovery of new scientific tests, based on detection of rRNA (made from the DNA of bacteria), which can detect both the type and the quantity of both living and dead bacteria in the gut; has led to a greater understanding of our gut microbiome.

Until recently, studies had difficulty in establishing which strains of bacteria may be linked to disorders, because they relied on culturing (growing) live bacteria; but the new 16s rRNA testing has made this so much easier. The tests are also much more accurate, as each rRNA is specific to particular bacteria and so we can now adjust our microbiome to health.

- **2015**

Current thinking, based on hundreds of research studies, is that there are three factors involved in autoimmunity:

> **1.** A **genetic** predisposition, (even though some of these genes may not be known, and the role of genes is minor) plus
> **2.** An **environmental trigger**(s) (including food) that instigates the immune response (and this is the main causal factor), plus

3. A breach of the intestinal wall barrier (**leaky gut**) which then allows the environmental trigger and the immune cells to inter-react. Leaky gut seems to precede all chronic and autoimmune disorders, and plays a major role in disease progression.

Allergies

Another extreme response to a trigger can be seen in allergies, where your immune system is hyper-reactive to something like pollen or particular foods. If you have an allergy to something you will probably know it, as you will get a rapid immune reaction to the trigger and it will be relatively severe. The good news is that healing inflammation, by removing triggers, together with restoring and feeding your gut microbiome, has also been found to reduce allergic reaction (see the chapter on solutions).

However, you may not be *allergic,* to the trigger but you may be *sensitive* to it. This is much more difficult to detect as it can take up to 72 hours for symptoms to develop, and the symptoms are less severe, but the sensitivity is nevertheless there. A good way to detect and eliminate food triggers is with an elimination diet, and we can read more about that later in the book in the chapter on Elimination Diets. One form of sensitivity is that to gluten, but in people without the genes for coeliac disease the reaction to the gluten is less severe.

Non- Coeliac gluten sensitivity

As we mentioned, about 1:100 people have coeliac disease, but gluten sensitivity is much more common, and has been associated with most of the same symptoms as those for coeliac disease. Not only that, it has also been associated with many other disorders in the body, including **migraines, ADD/ADHD, autism, neurodegenerative diseases (like Alzheimer's and Parkinson's** disease), autoimmune thyroid/hypothyroidism, autoimmune hepatitis, fibromyalgia, obesity and various skin problems.

The doctors can test for gliadin antibodies, which show that you are in danger of getting coeliac disease, so surely they can test for gluten sensitivity too? Most people would think so and would ask for this test to be done, however, most people with gluten sensitivity will find that these tests come back negative. Why?

Did your blood tests for gluten sensitivity come back negative?

The reason why the condition is so underdiagnosed by doctors and other healthcare providers, is that the primary test used by doctors to assess any reaction, at all, to gluten is the blood, is the test for gliadin antibodies, which they use to detect **coeliac disease**; but this may show a negative response (actually an extremely low count) because you do not have the genes which make the specific antibodies against *gliadin*, and this will result in the doctor telling you that you do not have a problem with gluten.

Although some people with gluten sensitivity *can* produce the same anti-gliadin IgG antibodies after eating wheat gluten that people with coeliac disease do, others will not produce antibodies at all, and so the test is not reliable as a diagnostic indicator.

There are now blood tests being developed to detect immune responses to the other peptides in gluten, and so this diagnosis will become easier, but until then the only way to *avoid* gluten sensitivity is by a gluten-free diet. However, to test for gluten sensitivity *before* embarking on a gluten free diet, the gold standard way to do this would be by using the **Elimination Diet** we talked about earlier. As you gradually introduce each thing back into your diet, you will see which, if any, triggers a reaction and produces symptoms (see chapter on Elimination Diets later in the book).

[We just read that the test for a reaction to gluten is by testing for gliadin antibodies. This is often done at a stage when you are suffering from quite severe symptoms of coeliac disease. In fact, autoimmune disorders are thought to be a continuum, and so if the condition is detected at an early stage, it may prevent the full blown journey to destruction of the microvilli by these antibodies.]

Unfortunately, after the 'negative' blood tests have been received, some doctors will then try to find *other* reasons for your symptoms. The good news is that you can discuss **gluten sensitivity** with your doctor and ask him/her to work together with you on a gluten free diet and assess your symptoms over a period of time as your diet changes. To do this, we need to be aware of the symptoms of gluten sensitivity.

Symptoms of non-coeliac gluten sensitivity

Although people with gluten sensitivity can have similar symptoms to coeliac disease and wheat allergies, those two disorders can be tested for and excluded; but the possibility of gluten sensitivity remains.

The symptoms for gluten sensitivity include **acid reflux (GERD), abdominal pain, bloating, burping, discomfort after eating, diarrhoea, constipation, foggy brain, headache, fatigue, joint and muscle pain, aching, numbness or tingling in arms and/or legs, eczema, rashes, depression, anxiety and anaemia.**

These symptoms occur in either hours or a few days after eating gluten, improve after gluten is withdrawn and re-occur in either hours or a few days after gluten is re-introduced into the diet.

The symptoms may not be recognised as signs of gluten sensitivity, especially if symptoms are those of anxiety or depression, which are not gut related; and so the only way to test for gluten sensitivity at the moment is to eliminate it from your diet for at least three weeks and see how you feel. You could then slowly integrate it back into your diet and see how you feel after a few days.

Could there be another culprit for 'gluten' sensitivity?

It may surprise you to learn that some of our food crops are sprayed with the herbicide Roundup ® (active ingredient is glyphosate) just before harvest; and that glyphosate can be found in the (non-organic) bread that we eat.

Glyphosate is considered to be non-toxic to humans, and other mammals, because humans do not have something called the shikimate pathway, an essential pathway in plants (and bacteria) which is destroyed by glyphosate.

Indeed, early toxicology studies suggested that glyphosate appeared to be non-toxic to humans and other mammals, but the studies were short (a three months test is industry standard, considered to be sufficient for this testing), and glyphosate was used in pure form rather than in combination with the additives that are always present in the herbicide products.

Two studies examining the toxicology of Roundup, showed that the additives to glyphosate are very toxic in themselves, and that they also increase the toxicity of glyphosate by an amount estimated to be at least 125-fold.

Recent research suggests that glyphosate also has many effects on the human body, even though it is considered to be non-toxic, and may cause the symptoms of gluten sensitivity in some people. This may be because glyphosate alters the balance between harmful and beneficial bacteria in the gut, causing a gut microbiome dysbiosis.

More information can be found on page 169.

Chronic disorders and autoimmunity as a continuum

It was the realisation that people could be sensitive to gluten that led to the theory that autoimmunity may not be a set disease, but a disorder that exists on a continuum. In other words, it gets gradually worse over time, in response to trigger(s), until it eventually becomes bad enough to be given a 'name', like type 2 diabetes or coeliac disease. The good news is that this immune response can be calmed down. Once you have supported your digestive system and healed your gut, through the measures listed in this book, molecular mimicry slows down and can stop altogether.

This is the fourth reason why I wanted to write this book, as I firmly believe, from all the scientific research that I have studied, that we can protect ourselves, and prevent the onset of chronic disease. (The other three reasons being, initially to help my family, the realisation that drugs for chronic disorders only treat symptoms, and that those drugs can cause long term harm). In addition, I was both surprised and delighted to find that some disorders can be reversed by making these easy changes.

Growing research is now proving that inflammation is created by our immune cells, and chronic inflammation happens because the trigger keeps on coming. When the gut microbiome is out of balance it can lead to chronic disorders. So we have a link between environmental triggers (including food), inflammation, and the gut.

- **2016**

It is now well established that Leaky gut is associated with many autoimmune disorders, including **multiple sclerosis, rheumatoid arthritis, irritable bowel disease** and **type 1 diabetes**; and also associated with **cancer** development and **allergies**, and that healing your gut may be the first step in healing your body.

Although this information is now well established in the scientific community, it hasn't filtered into the medical community to a great extent, which led to pioneers in the USA starting a whole new approach to diagnosis and treatment of chronic disorders, and it is called Functional Medicine. But how is this different to conventional medicine?

Functional Medicine

Functional medicine focuses on the *patient*, their story and their history, rather than focusing on the *disorder*. Patients are asked questions such as

- What is your lifestyle?
- What do you eat?
- How stressed are you?

It looks at potential **triggers** of the disorder or disorders which the patient is suffering from, and looks to find a solution by changing lifestyle and removing and avoiding the triggers of the disorder.

Ascertaining potential triggers in this way is not done in conventional medicine, as, in chronic 'disease', only the symptoms are treated usually, as there is no pharmaceutical 'cure'.

Busy doctors in the UK, who have barely enough time to even see all their patients, would, I am sure, like nothing better than to sit and chat with us, and, importantly, find a root cause for our condition rather than give us drugs which won't treat the root cause, and also may make the condition worse in the long term. It seems to be an essential part of preventing or curing these disorders, as triggers need to be found, but so far this is not happening in conventional medicine.

To summarise, functional medicine looks holistically at the person (their body, their diet and lifestyle and so on), whereas in conventional medicine we look only at specific symptoms, and diagnose a disorder of a *specific* organ, and then offer pharmaceutical drugs and/or surgery. Instead of looking at the person as a whole, we look at only a *part* of them, a *specific* organ within their body that seems to be having a problem. We even have specialists for different parts of our body; with gastroenterologists, cardiologists and so on.

This separatist approach to health has always baffled me, as our body works as a whole, and isn't isolated into its component parts. All of our 'systems', digestive, endocrine, cardiovascular, muscular and so on, 'talk' to each other, and are *constantly* aiming to achieve 'balance' (not too hot or too cold for example). This balance is called 'homeostasis', and so my approach to my research for this book was not to look at these different systems in isolation, as we do in conventional medicine, but to look at the whole picture; how your body works to achieve and maintain health, naturally, without a prescription.

In other words, to look at the wider picture, and think laterally, rather than focus narrowly on only one symptom of one organ, like, for example, the heart, or thyroid. I wanted to see if I could make connections between all sorts of different research, all specialising in different areas, and it turns out that they are there. I was joining the dots, to find the whole picture.

The other thing that we don't do in conventional medicine is consider how diet can affect health; and you may be surprised to know that although doctors receive training in pharmaceutical drugs and how they work in the body, they do not receive training in nutrition, other than get basic information such as vitamin C prevents scurvy. I doubt if many doctors see patients with scurvy, and for all other disorders they have their drug sheets.

I saw a programme on BBC One in November 2015, called **'Doctor in the House'**, with an inspirational medical doctor called Dr

Rangan Chatterjee, a GP in Oldham, who took time to stay with three families and help them to resolve their chronic disorders. He was recommending the measures I have found to be effective from my research (and have written about in this book so that you can do them too). It was really wonderful to see this approach to health, and hopefully there is a trend towards functional medicine in the UK too.

The good news is that **you can do much to help yourself**, working with your doctor if you have health problems of course. Your condition will have been diagnosed by your doctor, and so you can make the changes you need to improve it, put it into remission or even potentially reverse it and become healthy again. It is absolutely possible, and many medical doctors in the USA, who are functional medicine practitioners, are advocating this and seeing the results. However, with the help of this book, and many others, we are very fortunate here in the UK, as we can work together with our doctor, without any additional health charges; looking at potential triggers for chronic conditions which can be helped, and may be reversed in some cases.

Take home message

- The intestinal lining (epithelium), excluding the colon, has Tight Junctions which act like doors, usually closed but nevertheless doors.
- The opening of these Tight Junctions is highly regulated by your body, but the cholera toxin *Zot*, and human analogue (similar structure to *Zot*) zonulin can make products which also open the Tight Junctions. Any opening of the Tight Junctions, when they should still be closed, is called 'leaky gut'.
- Other environmental factors, like gliadin in wheat, can also cause these Tight Junctions to open when they shouldn't.

- Opening of the Tight Junctions, when they shouldn't be opened, means that large partly digested particles of food can get into your bloodstream. Your innate immune system then comes into contact with this partly digested food and recognises these particles as 'foreign'; starting an immune response, signally other immune cells to become involved, with associated inflammation.

- Repeated exposure to the triggers that cause the Tight Junctions to open, causes prolonged immune response with prolonged, chronic, inflammation, leading to chronic disorders (ones that last longer than three months).

- People with particular genetic susceptibility to getting certain disorders may have an increased hyper-immune response, leading to an autoimmune disorder, like coeliac disease. Others, who do not have those genes, but do possibly have other genes which react in a milder fashion, may have a sensitivity to certain triggers, like gluten.

- Some proteins in foods have a similar structure to human proteins (molecular mimicry) and, if a person has particular genes, this can lead to the attack, and potential destruction, of a specific organ (like the gut lining, or pancreatic cells, or the thyroid for example). When this happens the disorder is called an autoimmune disorder, as the body is attacking itself.

- Current medical response to chronic and autoimmune disorders includes medication to reduce the inflammation, treating the symptoms and not the root cause of the problem. Severe autoimmunity may also involve medication to suppress the immune system. This impacts on health as we need our immune system to fight harmful microbes and also to enable us to heal.

- Current medication to prevent inflammation may make the disorders worse over time, although other prescription drugs, like insulin for type 1 and possibly type 2 diabetes, and levothyroxine for hypothyroid disorders, are essential.
- There is a new approach to medicine called Functional Medicine, which looks holistically at the *whole* person, assessing their lifestyle to establish the **triggers** of their disorder and help to rectify that.

You may remember that earlier in the book, in the chapter on the benefits of having commensal bacteria, I alluded to the fact that your gut microbiome may somehow be linked to your mental health, as well as your physical health (for example by making serotonin which is the 'happy' hormone). Your gut and your brain are obviously not that close to each other physically, so how could your gut affect your mental health? Is there a link between your gut and your brain? It seems that there is! Let us look now at the gut-brain connection, which impacts not only on disorders like **Alzheimer's disease**, but on your **mood, anxiety, depression**, and even **food choices**!

Chapter Ten

The Gut-Brain Connection and Your Long Term Health (Key system Five)

If you cast your mind back to the forward of this book, I said that there are five key systems *in* your body that affect your long term health, and these are

- Your DNA
- Digestion
- Your immune system
- Your gut bacteria and
- Your brain

All of these interact with each other dynamically; adjusting their responses in order to keep us healthy (or try to). We have mentioned the first four earlier in the book, and now the fifth and final of those key body systems is your brain.

Gut-brain axis

The information about the gut that we have learned so far, and how it impacts on your long term health, would be amazing in itself, but when I tell you that your microbiome is also *directly* linked to your brain, via a gut-brain axis, where both brain and bacterial cells make products which can be 'read' and understood by each other, causing each other to react in certain ways, things get even more interesting!

Our digestive tract has its own (enteric) nervous system (which some are calling the 'gut brain'), which can send and receive impulses, record experiences and respond to emotions. Early in embryonic development, a bundle of neural tissue splits into two sections, with one section becoming the central nervous system (the brain and spinal cord) and the other becoming the enteric nervous system. These two systems are joined by a 'cable' of neurons called the vagus nerve. The 'gut brain' spreads throughout the gut tissue, including into the intestines, below the mucosal layer (where it is called the submucosal plexus). Here, the nerves are protected by glial cells that nourish the neurons, the immune cells, and also the "blood brain barrier" that keeps harmful substances away from important neurons in the brain. The 'gut brain' and main brain communicate with each other via nerve impulses along the vagus nerve, and also via messengers from immune cells (cytokines). (Interestingly, dysfunction of glial cells, and a compromised 'blood-brain' barrier, are seen in brain disorders like **Alzheimer's disease**).

In addition to the nervous systems, it is now recognised that the gut microbiome has a huge influence on the way we think; our **moods** and our responses, and this is why our microbiome, together with the enteric nervous system, is sometimes called a 'second brain'. Some bacteria make neurotransmitters, like serotonin (which makes us feel happy), and melatonin (which affects our sleep patterns), but evidence that the gut microbiome affects the brain and central nervous system *directly* has not been available until the past few years. This has now changed, and researchers studying the impact of the gut microbiome on brain and behaviour, have been able to make the connection using germ-free animals, probiotic supplementation, antibiotic administration, faecal transplantation studies and deliberate infections. It has now been established that our gut microbes can interact with the intestinal cells and the underlying nerves of the 'gut brain' (the enteric nervous system).

One example of how a gut microbiome can exert such an influence can be seen in one of the gut bacteria, *Lactobacillus rhamnosus*; which can influence its host, by directly altering GABA receptor expression in the central nervous system of mature healthy animals.

GABA is a neurotransmitter which regulates many physical and mental processes. Alterations in GABA receptor expression are seen in people with **anxiety, depression, and functional bowel disorders**; and these conditions often co-exist in the same patient. Treatment with a probiotic of *L. rhamnosus* could reverse this emotional behaviour, as can treatment with the probiotic *L. helveticus* (NS8).

This research also showed that these effects were not seen if the vagus nerve (the major nerve between the gut and the brain) was not functioning or did not exist, which suggests that the vagus nerve is the main communication pathway between the bacteria in the gut and the brain. However, there is now evidence for multiple pathways of communication from the intestinal microbiome to the brain, including via the immune system (cytokines), the brain-adrenal pathway and also the endocrine system (hormones). Probiotics **(*Lactobacillus*)** were shown to improve stress levels (in infant pups, caused by maternal separation of a few hours a day) and reduce increased levels of cortisol, triggered by an activated brain-adrenal pathway.

Epilepsy can also be associated with a GABA dysfunction, and so, although there has not been much research into this subject yet, it may be worth taking a probiotic containing *L. rhamnosus*, alongside medication for the epilepsy, sharing this information with relevant physicians. The 'For Every Day' probiotic by Optibac contains this strain.

It is well known that there are brain–gut interactions for the regulation of gut function in *both* healthy *and* diseased states. For example it was found that stressful life events could trigger bowel symptoms in patients with **Irritable bowel Syndrome (IBS).**

Stress also triggers the production of cortisol (a hormone with many functions, one of which is that it is a stress hormone) made by your brain, which, together with the pain signals received from your nerves, contributes to the inflammation involved in **chronic pain.**

Many of these known interactions were thought to be caused by the nervous system. For example, interruption of the nerve supply to the gut can prevent intestinal inflammation and diarrhoea caused by the toxins released by *Clostridium difficile* (*C. difficile)* bacteria in *C. difficile colitis.*

However, the role of the gut microbes (both commensal and pathogenic) in these interactions has now been recognized; and an imbalance in the number of different types of microbe (known as dysbiosis) is now know to be a major factor in human disorders such as **Inflammatory bowel disease**.

My research also led me to realise that people with **Autism Spectrum disorder (ASD)** also suffered from **anxiety** and **intestinal problems**; and also that they may have an abundance of *Clostridium difficile* bacteria. Could there be a link between these factors and **autism**? In 2000, autism was quite rare, with only 1:150 children, mainly boys, having it in the USA. In 2010 that rose to 1 in 68.

Children with ASD also experience high rates of **anxiety**, a sensitivity to sensory stimuli, and **gastrointestinal (GI) problems**, but the link between these symptoms and ASD were not examined until 2013; when 2973 children with ASD enrolled in the Autism Treatment Network (ages 2-17 years, 81.6 % male). The results indicate that anxiety, sensory over-responsivity and **GI problems** and ASD may have a common underlying root cause.

As we have just read, there may be links between the cause of **anxiety, gut problems** and **depression** in **ASD,** and so could the microbiome have an effect on ASD? Also what were the links between dysbiosis of the gut microbiome in ASD and anxiety and depression (if any)? I started my research. I needed to see if I could join the dots between anxiety, gut dysbiosis, depression, and, possibly, ASD.

Was there a link? One possibility comes from the food that we eat, or rather herbicide on the food, and this herbicide is glyphosate, used on genetically modified crops in areas of the world. Europe, so far, has ruled against these crops, although recent legislation allows each member state to make their own choice on the matter. Wales and Scotland will not be growing GM crops, but at the time of writing, England is not joining them. As mentioned earlier, in the section on gluten sensitivity, recent studies reveal that glyphosate may not be as harmless as has been suggested, and, together with aluminium, is linked to many neurological diseases, including **autism, depression, dementia, anxiety disorder** and **Parkinson's disease**. Recent studies show how glyphosate and aluminium, working together, can cause neurological damage.

The difficulty in establishing cause and effect between gut microbes and diseases outside of the gut.

Over the years there has been very little research to show links between gut microbes and chronic disease, as the research into gut bacteria has been very difficult, relying on culturing the bacterial cells to identify them, but many of the gut bacteria cannot be cultured outside of the body.

However, developments in science now means that the rRNA of bacteria (a product of DNA inside the bacterial cell) can be detected, even in dead bacteria. We no longer need to have cultures to show which bacteria are in the gut, and both the type and quantity of particular bacteria can now be assessed from faecal samples.

This contributed to research in 2013 which showed that an abundance of particular bacterial products in the bloodstream of offspring could influence host behaviour in **ASD**. There were also links between **ASD** and maternal immune activation (MIA), immune system interactions, and **increased permeability** of the gut.

This interested me, as high proportions of autistic children suffer from **gastrointestinal (GI) disorders**; implying, from what we have already read, a link between **autism** and abnormalities in the gut microbiome.

We have read that the microbiome has a major impact on our health, and that an imbalance in the types of bacteria, and other microbes like yeasts, can result in chronic disorders. There has now been increasing evidence to support this, from the gut microbiome bacterial rRNA sequencing analyses mentioned above, which indicates that disturbances in both the composition and diversity of the gut microbiome are indeed associated with various disease conditions.

However microbiome-level studies on autism are limited, and mostly focused on pathogenic bacteria. Several studies have reported an increased administration of oral antibiotics to autistic children during the first three years of life which would certainly have changed their microbiome diversity, but many children take antibiotics and don't get autism.

It is also known that lipopolysaccharide (LPS) (on the cell walls of gut bacteria) can induce inflammation in the brain, increasing permeability of the blood-brain barrier which, in turn, allows an accumulation of high levels of mercury in the brain, which may aggravate ASD symptoms.

Studies to assess the amount of mercury in children with autism, compared to those without autism, showed that the children with autism had lower levels of mercury in their first cut baby hair. This lower level of mercury may be due to a decreased ability to excrete it.

To date, there is very little research to investigate associations between antibiotics, mercury, gut disorders, anxiety, the gut microbiome and autism spectrum disorder, but, in my opinion, it warrants further research.

Breaking news!!

- Recent research has established that the core physiology (what is happening to the body on a physical, rather than behavioural, level) of autism spectrum disorder, has its root in inflammation, created by dysfunctional immune trigger(s), which is what we see in most chronic and autoimmune disorders.

- It has also been established that ASD occurs as a result of both inherited (genetic) factors and also environmental (epigenetic layer of information controlling the genes) factors. The next stage is to determine which environmental factors pose a risk of ASD.

- As research into this area of science expands rapidly, we are seeing growing evidence that an imbalance (dysbiosis) of the gut microbiome is associated with disorders both in the intestines and also throughout the body. The conclusion of an in-depth study in 2015 was that there is huge potential for manipulating the microbiome to sustain, improve, or restore the microbiome in individuals who are either 'at risk' of a chronic disorder or who are already suffering from a chronic disorder. In addition, changing the diet and microbiome of a pregnant mother may provide a balanced healthy microbiome in her offspring, with associated protection from chronic disorders.

- In addition to a balanced microbiome, it has been recently found that a gluten free diet, fed during pregnancy, changes the gut microbiome in both the mother and her offspring, and

111

reduces both inflammation in the gut and the incidence of **type 1 diabetes** in the baby.

The effect of stress on the gut microbiome

Some research also suggested a link between stress, its effect on the gut microbiome, and an increased vulnerability to disease. In infant rhesus monkeys separated from their mother, the stress experienced by the infants reduced some of their commensal bacteria, mainly *Lactobacilli*, and the reduction of these bacteria also increased their susceptibility to disease. The levels of the stress hormone cortisol rose (but could not explain the effects on the gut bacteria), and stress behaviour increased. The good news (putting aside for one moment the experiment on animals which is another ethical question) is that the levels of *Lactobacilli* were restored to normal levels after one week, and so the effects of the stress either seem to be temporary, or the bacterial balance may be restorable which, in turn, removes the stress. The relationship between stress and gut disorders has been well established, but it has now been shown that mental stress can destroy some gut bacteria; which, in turn, can impact on our health.

This restoration to normal levels interested me, and I looked further at the links between chronic disorders and probiotics. Could chronic disorders be temporary, and could people be restored to health by taking probiotics? As we just read, the levels of *Lactobacilli* were restored in the rhesus monkeys, and so their susceptibility to disease would have been reduced. Could taking probiotics restore bacteria to the gut that may, by taking antibiotics and eating foods that did not feed them very well, be at low levels in the microbiome? The answer is yes, and we read that an imbalance of gut microbes in our microbiome can cause disorders; so could restoring this balance remove the stress-associated disorders? We can read more about this in the chapter on solutions.

There are now new scientific tests, based on detection of rRNA (made from the DNA of bacteria), which can detect both the type and the quantity of both living and dead bacteria in the gut. Until recently, studies had difficulty in establishing which strains of bacteria may be linked to disorders, but the new 16s rRNA testing has made this so much easier as each rRNA is specific to particular bacteria and so we can now adjust our microbiome to health.

As with any test, it does have some limitations, but it seemed hopeful, particularly as mum and I had had such great results! I researched further because, although there was now a known link, the vagus nerve, between your gut and your brain, this did not explain how your brain might become inflamed, because your blood-brain-barrier protects you from this. Or at least it does if the barrier is working properly. I found a link between the gut and the brain which really surprised me, and it was called 'Leaky Brain'; with possible links to **Alzheimer's disease** and other disorders which we associate with the brain.

The Blood-Brain-Barrier can become 'leaky'.

Leaky Brain

Just as we read about **Leaky gut**, there is also something which is being called '**Leaky Brain**'. As we read earlier, your gut forms a barrier between its contents (the food that you eat and your gut microbiome) and the rest of your body; and something similar occurs between your blood supply (your circulatory system) and your brain. It is called the 'blood-brain barrier' (BBB).

The blood-brain barrier is a blood capillary membrane (endothelium) which is connected by Tight Junctions, not found in normal circulation. This membrane separates your circulating blood from the your brain, allowing water and small molecules like amino acids and glucose through, but preventing large molecules like toxins to get through. Does this sound familiar? It seemed to me to be acting in a very similar way to the gut lining, and, if that is the case, could those Tight Junctions also be affected by certain triggers? I researched further.

We read earlier that a protein found in the epithelium of the intestines is called Zonulin (ZO-1(zonula occluden protein-1)); and it is involved in both the structure and the function of Tight Junctions in patients with **coeliac disease.** I investigated **Alzheimer's disease** to see if there is a link to the blood brain barrier (BBB) and ZO-1 and found that there is, as zonulin also regulates the Tight Junctions in the brain. Both BBB damage and an imbalance of calcium in the brain have been linked to **Alzheimer's disease**; and so I wanted to see if I could join the dots, if they existed, between Leaky *gut* and **Alzheimer's disease**. What was happening to those Tight Junctions near the brain? To start, let us look at what **Alzheimer's disease** actually is.

Alzheimer's disease is a progressive neuro (nerve) degenerative disorder, which is characterised by an accumulation of an amyloid β (Aβ) peptide (part of a protein) in the central nervous system; which, together with other factors, leads to deposits of amyloid protein in the walls of the brain arteries. The protein is not usually deposited anywhere else in the body.

The accumulation of Aβ peptides is believed to be an early and causative event in cerebrovascular (cerebro = brain, vascular = blood vessels) alterations; and research has shown that alteration of permeability, and disruption of the blood brain barrier, are the major events of **Alzheimer's disease**.

Recent research suggests that taking a broad based probiotic may be beneficial in the *prevention* of brain disorders like **Alzheimer's disease.**

The mechanisms that underlie the changes in permeability are not clear yet, but we have read that environmental triggers are not always considered as possible causes in conventional medicine, and so we need much more research on this subject. Indeed, gluten may not even be considered as a possible cause for coeliac disease now if it wasn't for some amazing research by a lateral thinking few in the past. Could there be a trigger, or triggers that cause **Alzheimer's disease,** as they can cause **coeliac disease** and other chronic disorders? It seems possible, and **Alzheimer's disease** is being described by some as **'Diabetes type 3',** a form of diabetes mellitus that selectively afflicts the brain; and some of the drugs which are used to treat **type two diabetes mellitus** prevent many of the neurodegenerative effects seen in Alzheimer's disease.

So should we just take the drugs? Well type 2 diabetes is a lifestyle disease, and can be prevented and reversed by changes in your lifestyle without the need to take pharmaceutical drugs (with potentially damaging side effects); and so we go back to the drawing pin in the foot analogy. Do you want to remove the drawing pin in your foot or take drugs to help with the symptoms? The choice is always yours, but drugs do not cure either **type 2 diabetes** or **Alzheimer's disease**, which get progressively worse over time; whereas there is a possibility that lifestyle choices may prevent and possibly reverse them if you catch them in time.

It should be stressed here that people with **type 2 diabetes** won't necessarily get **Alzheimer's disease**. We are all unique, with unique DNA, and we all have unique lifestyles. What **type 2 diabetes** does indicate is that a person's body is out of balance and may have Leaky Gut. After reading recent research, it doesn't seem to be wildly impossible that Leaky Gut may be linked to a 'leaky brain', via Tight Junctions; the irregular opening of which, in response to a trigger or triggers (as we have already established) can cause chronic disease, particularly in people whose HLA genes react strongly to the trigger.

The exact triggers for **Alzheimer's disease** may not have been found yet, and the BBB does not work in *exactly* the same way as the intestinal epithelium; but if a simple trigger, or triggers, can prevent it, then, in my opinion, it is worthwhile investigating more. In the meantime, if we follow the protocols that prevent, help reduce, and even reverse chronic disorders (see the chapter on solutions), then, because of the fact that Tight Junctions are also found near the brain, it doesn't seem to be beyond the realms of possibility that it may also help prevent chronic disorder of the brain. Indeed, they may also help other brain disorders, like **epilepsy**, which is associated with GABA dysfunction. The probiotic *L. rhamnosus* has been found to reverse the anxiety and depression associated with GABA dysfunction and so, potentially, it may also help reduce those symptoms in people with **epilepsy**.

Brain disorders as a continuum

We now know that chronic disorders build over time, as the threshold of triggers and damage reaches such a point that your body can no longer keep up with the amount of healing and repair needed, and becomes unwell. In other words, they lie somewhere on a continuum, from just starting, with no symptoms, to a full blown chronic or autoimmune disorder like **type two diabetes** or **Alzheimer's disease**.

The main point of this book is to enable us all to prevent these disorders as much as possible, and so not get onto the continuum in the first place, and also to heal and reverse the ones we do have (unless the damage is too severe and has reached the point of no return). Even with severe damage however, it is *still* possible to prevent *other* chronic disorders from happening and reduce the severity of the ones we have. We will see in this book why our gut microbiome, and how we feed it, plays a major role in health and disease prevention; and because of the importance of food, I looked at this everyday necessity further.

My research into the connections between foods and our gut microbes made me wonder if our gut microbes could be actually influencing what we ate. I'm not suggesting that the gut microbes have some superior control over us, but they make neurotransmitters, which have an effect on our brain; and so could they have any other influence? If they could influence what we eat then that would help them thrive and survive, and so it seemed at least possible. I needed to know if that sugary cake you want to eat is driven by you or by your gut microbes! My research began!

Chapter Eleven

How Your Gut Microbiome Influences Your Food Choices, via the Gut-Brain Connection, and How This May Lead to Chronic Disorders

I had already found from research that gut microbes could influence your genes, by epigenetic control; and influence your emotions and wellbeing, by making neurotransmitters; and I wondered if the gut microbes could be exerting any other influence on you. Could they be influencing what you eat for example? It turned out that they can!

In earlier chapters we read that the type of food we eat, be it easily digested carbohydrates or slow release energy and fibre from some beans and plants, affects the *type* of bacteria and microbes that thrive optimally on those different types of food. For example, 'good' bacteria thrive optimally on soluble fibre from vegetables, whereas *Candida albicans*, a yeast, thrives very nicely on sugar and wants more! We also read that some of the microbes in your gut can produce toxins and various other chemicals, and an overload of *Candida* can certainly cause brain fog and other unpleasant symptoms. We should say here that this only happens if there is an *overgrowth* of *Candida*, which has happened because of bacteria in the gut being destroyed (by antibiotics, and by us not eating the vegetable fibre that they need to survive), leaving space for the *Candida* to spread along the gut. In other words, the microbes that survive and thrive are the ones we feed (and do not kill with antibiotics)!

What we *haven't* read up to now is that some of those toxins and chemicals produced by all gut microbes can influence both your **food choices** and your **behaviour**. But how? We must be in ultimate control, but when we think of some of our choices, be it eating too many cakes or eating junk food with poor nutritional value, maybe that gives us pause for thought? Is it really 'you' that wants the extra cake?

This sounds like science fiction, but recent research shows that your gut microbes influence eating *behaviour* and your dietary *choices* to favour particular nutrients they grow best on; rather than simply passively living off whatever food we choose to send their way.

We have read that different bacterial and other microbe species vary in the nutrients they need. Some prefer fat, others fibre, and others sugar, for example; but not only do they vie with each other for food, and to retain their 'niche', their place in your digestive tract, they may also want different foods to the ones which keep you healthy. Sugar is a prime example of this! In other words, some gut microbes have similar dietary goals to you, whereas others do not! The microbes are manipulative and fight for survival, which may give you the cravings you find so difficult to resist. **BUT!** The good news is that you can alter the composition of your gut microbes in only 24 hours! Feed the good bacteria which make you healthy and happy, and, by not eating things like sugar, you can also kill the microbes which make you crave sugar and other unhealthy things like alcohol, which is also a source of sugar for *Candida.* (Alcohol also contributes to leaky gut, but it only has a temporary effect!).

I mentioned that the microbes can change your eating *behaviour* and this may also be linked to your lifestyle choices, and so in the short term you will need to override those thoughts, make a healthy start, maybe some very simple exercises for just five minutes a day before meals, and within a very short time you can be on the road to health and happiness!

We read earlier that some bacteria (*Lactobacilli*) can alleviate **stress** (and so gut microbes can also impact on our **mood**). What I didn't understand was why the microbes were making these chemicals and how it might benefit them, as I didn't know that they were linked to your brain by your vagus nerve. Recent research, however, shows that they are indeed linked to the brain, but how does this link affect our food choices?

Recent studies, published in 2014, show that the microbes influence your **food choices** by altering the nerve signals in your vagus nerve, changing **taste receptors**, producing toxins to make you **feel bad**, and releasing chemical rewards to make you **feel good**. This influence results in you eating and drinking particular nutrients that the microbes grow best on!

Some of those influences can be to induce cravings, which can be a major problem for people who are alcohol dependent; and so could altering the gut microbiome of alcohol-dependent people help them to stop drinking? The answer seems to be YES!!

Recent research shows that those alcohol dependent people who struggled with alcohol cravings after giving up alcohol for a few weeks, had high intestinal permeability (leaky gut), and their scores of **depression, anxiety**, and **alcohol craving** remained increased, even when they had stopped drinking for more than two weeks. However, the alcohol dependent people with normal, or low, intestinal permeability did not get the alcohol cravings after withdrawal from alcohol for two weeks, and recovered completely for **depression** and **anxiety**.

Alcohol has been shown to temporarily cause leaky gut, but as all patients in the study drank alcohol, this did not seem to be the *only* trigger.

I suspected that these people may be suffering from gut dysbiosis (an imbalance in the diversity and numbers of their gut bacteria) and so I researched further. There have been few studies to research gut permeability in alcohol dependent humans, but one study observed a decrease in *Bifidobacterium* and *Lactobacillus* in the stool cultures of alcohol dependent people with liver damage compared with those of healthy controls.

The microbiome of these people was restored with the probiotics *Bifidobacterium bifidum* and *Lactobacillus plantarum 8PA3*, and patients with alcohol-induced liver injury showed a greater improvement after taking these probiotics, rather than standard therapy alone.

In addition to restoring the gut lining, other studies show that probiotics also have an effect on the immune system, reducing inflammation by producing anti-inflammatory cytokines, which may also help people with liver damage.

Alcohol also affects the levels of **ghrelin** in your body, and we know that drinking alcohol increases appetite (one of the functions of ghrelin), but increased ghrelin levels can also increase alcohol craving in alcoholics.

In the chapter on the microbiome, we see how **ghrelin** has another function, as well as increasing appetite, and levels of ghrelin in your body also increase if you have inflammation in your gut lining. In alcoholics, this could be the reason for the increased levels of ghrelin seen. You can read more about ghrelin in the next chapter.

My personal opinion is that if a change to your gut microbiome can reduce cravings for alcohol, then it may also help people with **cravings** for **nicotine,** and **sugar**, and so may be worth considering as a potential therapy for all cravings.

Is your gut microbiome a second brain?

Some people are actually calling the gut microbiome a 'second brain', but, although the microbes certainly have a huge influence on you, it is *you* that is in ultimate control; and as we already mentioned, one of the major differences between your brain and your microbiome is that your microbiome changes regularly; mainly in response to environmental causes, and, in particular, in response to diet and lifestyle. It may also change for the better after taking probiotics, particularly after a course of antibiotics, which may have killed many of the 'good' bacteria in your gut.

Like everything else, when you have the information, you can make informed choices. If you change your microbiome you may not need 'willpower', as the microbes that 'want' the bad stuff (that makes you unwell) simply won't be exerting an influence any more. Not only that, the microbes that make you feel great, and influence you to eat the good stuff that makes you healthy and happy (in other words, vegetables, so your mum was right all along!!), will be your major influence. No fighting against cravings, no struggling with willpower, (although sometimes your 'memory buttons' may make you think that you still like or want something, but that is just a memory flashback so ignore it!). Sounds good!

Like everything else in life though, you have to take an active part if you want to achieve a successful outcome. As we read earlier, some bacteria can be destroyed much more easily than others, and this can result in an imbalance of microbes in your gut, with a decrease in 'good' bacteria and an increase in microbes like *Candida* yeast in your microbiome (with a resulting influence on you to eat things like sugar). By removing processed sugar, and simple carbohydrates (which are rapidly converted to glucose) from your diet, your gut microbiome gets the chance to return to a healthy balance, and so you need to help it! The reason, I now realise, that we call the microbes 'bad' isn't because they are bad *per se* (they are, after all, just trying to survive) but because the food that they want us to eat, although great for them, may not be best for your health. There is a conflict of interest!

- *But, there is no need to be concerned! This biggest thing to remember here is that microbes have an incredibly short lifespan (some replicate in twenty minutes) and the microbiome can be manipulated easily, as we read earlier, by prebiotics, probiotics, antibiotics, faecal transplants, and dietary changes. These changes offer a hope for seemingly epidemic proportions of obesity, 'unhealthy eating', and most chronic disorders; and your microbiome can be changed in only 24 hours!*

The other good news is that it is relatively easy to get rid of the 'bad' microbes in your gut, which are making you obese or unhealthy or depressed, and replace them with more 'good' bacteria, which make you healthy and happy. You can achieve a healthy body, healthy weight, healthy wellbeing and healthy mind, and this book will give you the tools to do it in the chapter on solutions.

What we should remember though is how helpful our gut microbiome is to us, and how it can keep us healthy and happy. For example, one of the commensal bacteria in the gut, *Bacteroides fragilis* can protect animals from **colitis** caused by *Helicobacter hepaticus*, (a commensal bacterium which can become pathogenic) by producing polysaccharide A (PSA). In fact, if PSA is not produced by *B. fragilis,* there is an increase in *Helicobacter hepaticus* colonisation, which leads to disease and inflammation of the colon. In other words, PSA, produced by a gut bacterium, protects us from inflammatory disease by preventing an excess of colonisation by potentially harmful microbes.

Put simply, the balance between the numbers and diversity of these different microbes is linked to the critical balance between health and disease.

Gut bacteria can directly influence gut balance (homeostasis) and health in other ways too; for example by regulating the rippling effect that moves your food throughout your digestive system, and also by influencing the immune response in the gut; for example, *Lactobacillus farciminis* was shown to release nitric oxide in the colon, which has an anti-inflammatory effect.

We mentioned a hormone called ghrelin, in the chapter on the digestive tract, which makes you feel hungry, but which also has another function as it responds to inflammation in your gut. The counter hormone to ghrelin is leptin, and this tells you when you feel full. Leptin also responds to inflammation in the gut, but in the opposite way to ghrelin. The reason I mention this is because it is now known that leptin is actually made in your adipose tissue. In other words, it is made in the layer of fat beneath your skin. This revelation made researchers take a closer look at your fat cells, and the results were surprising! In fact, your fat cells are now considered to be another endocrine organ, which produces and releases hormones! Could this be linked to chronic disorders? The answer was yes! I needed to know more about our fat cells!!

Take home message

- You are still in ultimate control. We just need to be aware that it may not be 'you' that wants the unhealthy product. If we take a moment to think about that, it actually makes sense. Why would your body want you to eat or drink something that made it unhealthy, when it is constantly aiming to restore balance and achieve health?

Chapter Twelve

Fat - A New Endocrine Organ is discovered

One new thing to emerge from recent research, when considering chronic disorders, diet, and the food that we eat; and especially links to **obesity**, are your fat cells. As we read earlier, human fat is mainly stored just beneath the skin and is called adipose tissue, but we also store fat around organs and muscle (this is why you can't see muscle definition if you are overweight). We knew that our body stores excess nutrients as fat for an energy source for when food is in short supply, but we did not know that adipose tissue actually produces hormones! It actually functions like an endocrine organ, such as thyroid, in that it secretes hormones into the bloodstream, and the hormone that it secretes is leptin. Let us take a closer look at fat!

Fat – Adipose tissue

We briefly mentioned hormones in our chapter on the digestive tract, as being involved in the digestion and absorption of our food, but hormones can have more than one function. For example, two hormones that are involved in us having enough food for energy play a major part in the digestive process, and these are ghrelin and leptin, and these hormones are also involved in immune responses. But why would they have these two functions?

It seems odd at first, but if we remind ourselves that most harmful microbes reach us via the food and drink that we ingest, it may not be so surprising. To explain further, let's look firstly at ghrelin and leptin in more detail.

Leptin and Ghrelin – the 'full' and 'hunger' hormones

Leptin and ghrelin are two hormones that are known to have a major influence on energy balance. Leptin influences long-term regulation of your energy balance, suppressing your food intake and inducing weight loss. As well as being made by your fat cells, leptin is thought to be a product of what some call your 'obesity gene', and it is your 'feel full' hormone; whereas ghrelin makes you feel hungry.

Ghrelin

Ghrelin is your 'hunger' hormone, which kicks in when you haven't eaten. Hormones, once released, always travel to another area of your body to make things happen. In this case, the hormone ghrelin is made mainly by your stomach and travels via your bloodstream to your brain, resulting in a strong urge to eat.

Ghrelin is also made by immune T cells, and its other function is to inhibit inflammation in the gut.

Already here I could see a possible connection between inflammation in the gut and a desire to eat. If ghrelin inhibits gut inflammation, but also increases hunger, the dots seem to be joining.

The 'bad' microbes in your gut, which produce toxic lipopolysaccharides (LPS), are one cause of inflammation in the gut that the ghrelin attempts to remove. These microbes also fight the hormone ghrelin and try to knock it out, and so there is a constant battle between them, especially if the microbiome is out of balance and potentially 'bad' microbes dominate.

When you have eaten, ghrelin levels fall, and leptin sends a message to your brain telling it that you have had enough food and that your fat reserves are topped up again, and so not to eat any more.

Leptin

Leptin is also a hormone, and is made mainly in fat cells (white adipose tissue). Its main function is the opposite of ghrelin i.e. it stops feelings of hunger. Leptin, like ghrelin, is also made by your immune T cells, and in this capacity as a cytokine (an immune messenger, signalling other immune cells to become active); but rather than *reducing* inflammation (like ghrelin) leptin *increases* inflammation, by producing cytokines which start an immune response. So you have one hormone, ghrelin, which is anti-inflammatory and another hormone, leptin, with is pro-inflammatory. It isn't difficult to see why these need to be in balance!

If your leptin signalling is working properly, when your fat stores are full they cause a surge in your leptin levels, which signals your brain to stop feeling hungry and stop eating. It also directs your brain to stop storing fat and to start burning some excess fat off.

In people who suffer from obesity, leptin (which tells you to stop eating) is *increased*, whereas the level of ghrelin is decreased, but the leptin does not suppress appetite. The reason for this is because **obese** people are **leptin-resistant**, but what is leptin-resistance? Well, you become leptin-resistant (and also insulin-resistant) by continuous overexposure to, and high levels of, the hormone (in this case, leptin); which results in your body's systems becoming exhausted and not working properly. The end result is that your body does not 'hear' the signal; and we call this 'resistance'.

The only known way to re-establish normal leptin (and insulin) signalling is to prevent those surges, and the only known way to do that is via a healthy diet, with plenty of vegetables and whole foods, as we read earlier. *These changes in diet can change your health and reverse chronic disorders like* **obesity** *and* **Type II diabetes**.

One theory for rising levels of obesity in western populations is that the body's mechanisms for controlling appetite evolved to match ancestral diets with more low-energy plant foods. This may explain why, if we eat fibre-rich vegetables, like beans, we feel full, even though they may not have as many calories as other foods. It may also explain why we can eat lots of non-fibrous foods without feeling full. For example, if one of the main triggers for leptin is the short chain fatty acids produced, from fibre, by our gut bacteria; and we don't eat very much fibre, then the 'feel full' signals will not happen as quickly. In that scenario, ghrelin tells us to keep eating. Of course, what our body means by the ghrelin signal is to eat more fibre, but in a 'Western diet' we may eat pizza or cake instead!

We just read that fat cells have a function, other than storage of fat for energy (one being the production of the hormone leptin), and this has revolutionized our thinking. In fact, the entire understanding of the endocrine system (the collection of glands, like the pancreas and thyroid, which secrete hormones directly into the blood system, rather than ducts, to be carried towards a distant target organ, like the brain) has had to be re-assessed.

This new understanding of the function of fat cells means that stored fat is actually a metabolic organ, making and expressing hormones, much like your thyroid gland or adrenal glands (and so can have **a** major impact on our health if we have too much, *or too little*, stored fat).

In summary, fat cells:

- Store fat for use by the body in times of low food supply, and
- Produce the hormone leptin, which, together with ghrelin, regulates our hungry/full signals.

However, what interests us for the purposes of this book, is that these two hormones **leptin and ghrelin, are also involved in your immune responses in your gut** (and, as we read, immune responses can lead to chronic inflammation and chronic disorders).

Fat cells also store toxins

Fat cells also store other things and these include toxins which your body wants to remove out of circulation. In other words your body wants to contain them so that they cannot do you harm. This happens if your body isn't excreting the toxins through the normal channels of sweat, urine and so on quickly enough. When fat is released, during times of starvation or when dieting, these toxins are also released and so you can feel temporarily unwell (until the toxins are eliminated out of the body) but once they have gone you will be rid of them forever, so that is good news!. Another storage area for toxins is joints, and this can lead to pain in your joints. The answer is simple really, and that is to avoid toxins wherever possible, and to help the body eliminate them if you do have them. We will read more about this later in the book in the chapter on Elimination Diets, which are the gold standard for determining your triggers of your chronic disorder(s).

Take home message

- Fat cells make a hormone called leptin, which is pro-inflammatory (it starts an immune response).
- Leptin works together with ghrelin to control your 'full/hungry' responses and resulting food intake, but ghrelin, as well as making you feel hungry, also reduces inflammation in your gut.
- It isn't difficult to see how a trigger which causes gut inflammation can then also cause an increase in the hormone ghrelin, which, in turn, increases your appetite. If you keep eating, in response to the huge mental urge created by the ghrelin hormone, then more and more leptin will be produced, as fat cells fill and fill. One can also see how this may be linked to obesity in some way, both from a perspective of over-eating and also because of the surge in

leptin caused by the over-eating, which may also lead to leptin-resistance.

• Both ghrelin and leptin have a very powerful effect on your body, as they target your brain directly, and the urge to eat, in response to ghrelin, is exceedingly difficult to override. However, as leptin-resistance means that your brain cannot 'hear' the message from your leptin that you have eaten enough, it is also easy to see why this is linked to obesity. The good news is that leptin-resistance (just like insulin-resistance) is reversible, when changes are made to your diet.

So the dots are joining. We have read so far that inflammation of the gut lining, and opening of Tight Junctions as a result of triggers, which include some 'food' can result in an ongoing immune response, resulting in chronic inflammation in some parts of the body, and brain.

We also read that some hormones have two functions, for example ghrelin is involved in both hunger and reducing inflammation in the gut; and leptin reduces hunger.

Leptin, produced by adipose tissue (fat cells), can, when there is a constant production of ghrelin (in response to the inflamed gut), go into overdrive, as it keeps trying to tell the brain that the fat cells are full and we don't need to eat any more food; resulting in the **leptin resistance** seen in **obesity**.

Throughout all of this there is also a link to the gut microbiome, which, when out of balance, can cause us to want to eat things which make us unhealthy. An unbalanced gut microbiome also affects our health and wellbeing as we may be deficient in those bacteria which produce things we need, for example some vitamins. Deficiencies of some bacteria can also affect our mental health as some produce serotonin, the happy hormone, the lack of which can cause anxiety and depression

Although we have been able to join many dots so far, it all comes back to getting your body back in balance, and the first step to achieve this is with a balanced healthy microbiome, and a healthy gut. In other words, heal your gut and you heal your body. How do we get a healthy microbiome compared to an unhealthy microbiome? That's easy. You get the one you feed.

We have been looking at the potential problems and reasons why we get chronic disorder, but now let us look at the solutions!

Chapter Thirteen

The Solutions to Your Long Term Health (Your Sixth 'Key System') and Your Five-Step Plan

We have mentioned the five key systems in your body that are major players in your long term health (DNA, digestion, immune system, gut bacteria, and your brain); and we have read how they interact dynamically with each other. We also read that various *environmental* factors, like diet, can have a major impact on those systems. As your diet, environment, lifestyle and even state or mindfulness can have a *major* effect on your long term health, and interact with **all** your key health systems, I am going to call this group, and the information included in this chapter, your '**sixth key system**', even though it is *outside* of your body. For example, your diet actually interacts with your DNA, which then turns your genes on or off (see the chapter on DNA); and other environmental factors, like availability of food during development, can change your gut bacteria, which then either influence either long term health, or disease. The good news is that we learned that we can make the changes needed for our health; and that is what we are talking about in this chapter. The solutions.

The solutions consist of some easy steps and some small changes in your life, using a five-step plan which is:

Five-step plan

1. Re-inoculating your gut microbiome (as some essential bacteria are killed off with antibiotics and other things that you may have taken).

2.   Feeding the healthy microbiome, and taking supplements where needed.
3.   Removing food triggers to restore your gut to health.
4.   Avoiding non-food triggers where possible.
5.   Taking steps to get enough sleep and exercise, and manage stress.

Let us look at these in more detail, starting with gaining a new healthy microbiome! The reason why we are looking at gaining and feeding a healthy balance microbiome is because the starting point for most chronic disorders is a dysbiosis in the gut. In other words having a gut microbiome that is out of balance, but why is this important? Let us remind ourselves of why a balanced gut microbiome might be beneficial.

Firstly, different bacteria produce different enzymes, which produce different products (like butyrate and vitamins), all of which are needed by your body. Some bacteria also make neurotransmitters which affect your wellbeing and your thought processes; whereas others, if out of balance, produce levels of toxins which, in excess, make you feel bad (either mentally or physically)

Secondly, gut bacteria have a relationship with your immune system, which lies below the mucosal layer in your intestines. Some bacteria can reduce inflammation, whereas others can increase it. As all chronic disorders have chronic inflammation, it makes sense to reduce the bacteria which can cause this increase in inflammation or make it worse.

Thirdly, your gut bacteria also have a relationship with fat cells (adipose layer) most of which is directly under your skin, although some is around your organs; and some bacteria promote fat storage, whereas others don't. In addition to this, inflammation created in your gut also has a relationship with your adipose tissue, as these fat cells also produce leptin, a hormone which promotes inflammation (we read about leptin and ghrelin earlier, the 'full' and 'hungry' hormones, which have more than one function).

Dysbiosis is also linked to Leaky Gut. This is when the mucosal layer of the intestine lining, and Tight Junctions, have been breached, allowing the underlying immune cells to come into contact with the *contents* of your intestine (broken down food and bacteria), none of which are *self,* and so Leaky Gut creates an immune response with associated inflammation. However, some bacteria help to heal Leaky Gut.

We also read earlier that certain things can manipulate your gut microbiome for the *better*, leading to a **healthier body and mind**. Let us look at each of these, reminding us first of what they are:

- Prebiotics (eating for health) and dietary changes
- Probiotics (restoring your gut microbiome), and their effect on specific diseases; antibiotics; faecal transplants,
- Avoid food triggers, and non-food triggers of your disorder
- Stress (you learn how to stop it exerting a control over you) and
- Sleep (you need this to heal your body and mind)
- Supplements that may be helpful.

You notice that I mention the things which may cause you problems (triggers of chronic disorders), BUT!! Although there *are* triggers, there are also things you can do to avoid them and also prevent and even reverse the *effects* of these triggers, and so you should not be despondent or feel overwhelmed. There are solutions and they are easy!

Breaking news!

Finally, exciting new research involving hundreds of people, published in November 2015, has proven that eating for your microbiome can change the microbes in your gut, and that this can reduce your chances of getting chronic disorders. The research showed that we do not all respond in the same way to the same food. For example, some people had raised blood glucose after eating bananas, while others did not; and this was linked to the different bacteria that they had in their gut. After a few days of making a change in their diet, the researchers found that the gut microbiome of the people in the study also changed! Exciting stuff! All of the research I have read also shows this, but to have one piece of research, specifically looking at people eating in their normal way, eating what they normally ate, looking at the times of day that they ate, their lifestyle and their environment, supports all of the findings in this book.

In summary, eat mainly vegetables, with a little organic meat or fish in moderation if you wish to, and some fruits. Eat a variety of vegetables, with some nuts and seeds, in order to get all the nutrients, phytonutrients and protein that you need. Easy! Remember that the changes in our diet over the last sixty years have been motivated by the profits of big business rather than health!

Your symptoms

O.K., before we get started there is something you need to do first, and that is to make a note of all of your symptoms. I mention this in the elimination diet in chapter fifteen, but I mention it here as we need to see how we are progressing so that we can see how we have improved; and so keep a daily or weekly record, depending on how you feel. As well as noting your symptoms, it may also be useful to have your antibody levels checked if this is possible. For example, some people may have the autoimmune version of hypothyroidism (where the body doesn't produce enough thyroid hormone) called Hashimoto's thyroiditis, and produce TPO and TG antibodies, which attack their own thyroid gland; and these can be raised for ten years before their TSH test (which indicates problems with the thyroid gland) shows any changes (source: *'Reversing Hashimoto's: Nutrition and Beyond'; webinar, Dr Izabella Wentz, 24 March 2016)*. People may be suffering from anxiety, depression, IBS and chronic fatigue, and be given medication for those symptoms, but the root cause may lie with their thyroid gland; however, with a normal TSH, most doctors will not investigate further. People with Graves' disease (autoimmune hyperthyroidism, where the thyroid produces too much thyroid hormone) will also have raised antibodies (source: *Dr Amy Myers MD)*

The antibody test is useful for three things. One, it confirms why you are feeling that something isn't quite right, in spite of other tests (like the TSH) that tell you everything is fine; two, the antibody levels, if raised, need to be brought back down to at least remission levels (where they no longer attack your thyroid gland in this example); and three, they show, together with your symptoms (that you are recording) that the changes you are making are working for you.

It is very important to say here that not everyone with hypothyroidism or hyperthyroidism produces antibodies against their own organs, but it is worth checking in my opinion. For those of us who don't produce antibodies, or who are unable to have the tests for antibodies done, the record of symptoms is perfectly fine and will be a good record of your improvement. (TPO = Thyroid peroxidase antibodies; TG = Thyroglobulin Antibodies; TSH = Thyroid Stimulating Hormone).

Probiotics and restoring your gut microbiome to health

We read in the chapter on probiotics that some strains of bacteria are destroyed more easily than others by antibiotics, and so these are the ones which we usually want to replace by taking probiotics. As we read, there are different qualities of probiotic so are they all as good as each other?

136

Are all Probiotics as good as each other?

The short answer to that is no, but I will explain a little bit about them first.

Most probiotic bacteria were isolated originally from healthy humans, as these were considered to be safe for human consumption (the first example being *Tissier*, who, we read earlier, treated infants suffering from diarrhoea with probiotics, from human breast milk, with positive results). Some are still produced from animal products although vegan ones are also available. I will explain more when I give you information about specific probiotics as we read through this section.

As we read earlier, probiotics belong to a specific genus or family, like Lactobacillus, and within each genus, or family are particular species, like *rhamnosus*. Finally, they are divided further into particular strains, and these are often denoted with a particular reference number, like, for example, Rosell-11.

Why are the probiotics divided into all of these different categories? Well the *genus* and *species* sort the bacteria by their specific properties (like producing butyrate or lactic acid for example); and also where they settle in different parts of the body, and different parts of the colon (and exert their effects there); and the *strain*, with its reference number, indicates the volume of research it has been involved in. For example, L. acidophilus is a 'good' probiotic *species* in general, but the specific *strains* such as NCFM® or Rosell-52 tells us which *types* of acidophilus were clinically tested in particular situations (for example, testing the effectiveness of a particular strain in patients with **eczema**).

However, although different bacterial species and strains have unique properties, many of their functions also overlap, and so don't be too anxious if you cannot find a particular *strain* of probiotic to purchase. As research expands into this area, more and more strains

137

will become available. As we mentioned earlier, you only have four different phyla of bacteria in your gut (in the main), and we each have a variety of different species within those phyla. If those species varied that much in function we would not have that variety as we would not survive if we didn't have specific ones, and so that is why I say not to worry too much about specific species; however, some species may be more *beneficial* than others in particular situations (for example if you have certain genes which dispose you to a particular chronic disorder), but you can change your microbiome, almost overnight, so that is not a problem either!

Once probiotics have been grown, they are tested to ensure that the live bacteria can reach the gut without being destroyed along the way (for example by the stomach acid).

The gold standard for this testing results in pharmaceutical grade probiotics, but not all probiotics that are available for purchase are pharmaceutical grade. They may not have passed all the rigorous tests which ensure that they can reach the gut without being destroyed and are therefore effective. It is important to check where the probiotics come from for this reason. There will be several to choose from I am sure, but I will tell you about the ones I have tried as I have checked these out, and they are by a company called Optibac. My opinion is my own, and it is unbiased. I do not have any association with this company, nor do I receive any financial rewards from them! The probiotics work for me and so this is the only reason why I am sharing the information with you now.

Optibac use a company called **Lallemand Health Solutions**, who make pharmaceutical grade products. The ones I bought for my mum and myself (I mentioned this in the chapter on my mum) were the **Optibac 'For Every Day'**. I started with the **extra strength** ones, and then tried the 'For Every Day' ones. Other probiotics are available, but I bought the 'For Every Day' ones because it is a broad based probiotic, with several strains, which offer different benefits, and these strains were chosen by the company because of very good scientific evidence which shows that those particular strains have a beneficial effect.

Other strains of probiotic may suit you better, and, like most things, it is a case of trial and error. (I tried other ones first, but they didn't seem to help at all). We have stayed with Optibac because their probiotics helped my mum both mentally and physically, whereas other brands didn't. This may not be the same for you of course, we are all different. I continue to use them because my allergic responses have reduced massively, and I rarely get colds. In other words, my immune system is in balance and is working well.

I have noticed that my allergic rhinitis is much better when I take Optibac 'Every Day Extra Strength', rather than just the 'Every Day' ones. This may be because there are simply more live bacteria in the extra strength capsules, but it may also be because the strain of Lactobacillus in the Extra Strength capsules is *L. acidophilus NCFM®*, whereas the strain in the Every Day capsules is L. *acidophilus Rosell-52*. The latter is a well-researched strain of acidophilus, found to adhere well to the gut lining, but the former, when taken together with *Bifidobacterium lactis Bl-04* (also in the Extra Strength probiotic) can help alleviate allergic rhinitis.

How many live bacteria should there be in a probiotic?

There is no fixed dosage and so the numbers can vary, but, as a guide, you should be looking at those with several to many billions of live bacteria. For example, the Optibac 'For Every Day' probiotics have 5 billion live bacteria, and Optibac 'For Every Day Extra Strength' probiotics contain 20 billion live bacteria.

Probiotics – A Miracle Cure?

The reason I mention this is because probiotics alone, no matter how helpful they are, are *not* miracle cures. Life is *never* as **simple as** 'take a tablet and everything will be fine', and taking a probiotic is no different.

The thing to bear in mind is that the microbes in our gut are *commensal*. They work *with* us. If they actually had the *power* to reduce excess fat to such a degree that they could cure **obesity**, for example, they wouldn't be commensal anymore they would be pathogenic! They would have the power to control you. They wouldn't 'know' when you were just the right healthy weight, they would keep on taking your nutrients. Be thankful that a probiotic cannot control your body!

There has been much research to try and find the miracle probiotic. The cure. This is, of course, because someone wants to market it as a 'cure' and make lots of money from it. It isn't going to happen. Some probiotic strains may benefit you more than others, but you also need to make a few changes to help them keep you healthy. I have made a few changes, as well as taking probiotics, and these are all mentioned below.

Probiotics and Leaky gut

We read earlier that your microbiome, among other things, keeps your gut healthy, by producing things like butyrate, and also by crowding out harmful bacteria. This is why probiotics can be helpful, as antibiotics destroy some of the strains in the gut (like *lactobacilli and bifida*) more easily than others (like *bacteroides*), and so taking a probiotic which contains some of these bacterial strains can replace the ones you have lost, and bring your gut back into (healthy) balance.

As I just mentioned however, if you keep eating and drinking harmful triggers, which damage your gut and lead to leaky gut, you are in a vicious circle of heal-attack-heal-attack. This is why you need to:

1. Heal your gut
2. Remove the triggers of damage

Preferably at the same time.

Certain Strains of Probiotic Bacteria are Effective in Treating Disease

As we read earlier, it used to be much more difficult to detect which bacteria actually lived in the gut, as the tests relied on them being cultured (grown) in a laboratory from a faecal specimen taken from you. However many of the gut bacteria could not survive outside of the body and so could not be detected. This has now changed as we can detect the DNA of the different bacterial strains from a sample (usually faeces), even if they are no longer alive.

In addition to the new 16s rRNA scientific advances enabling us to identify the bacteria, there have also been clinical trials to evaluate the effects of probiotics on certain symptoms of gut disorders, where they have been shown to both enhance gut barrier function and inhibit pathogen binding.

You may find it helpful to have information from some of these studies, in relation to particular disorders and the strains they used in the research, and so I will include some of this here. However, many different strains of a particular species often overlap with their function, (in other words they do the same thing in our body, like, for example, produce butyrate) and so please remember that before you become too concerned about finding particular strains in your choice of probiotic.

The good news is that altering your gut microbiome composition, by taking probiotics, and feeding it with healthy prebiotic food, results in your new microbiome remaining stable, as long as you stick with the healthy way of eating! Studies certainly show that our gut microbiome remains stable while ever we are taking a broad based probiotic (with sufficient numbers of live bacteria in it – see Optibac for suggestions of the numbers needed, but they range from 5 billion to 20 billion live bacteria per capsule).

Probiotics and Hashimoto's Thyroiditis (Autoimmune Hypothyroidism)

Dr Isabella Wentz, who has studied **Hashimoto's Thyroiditis** extensively, found that people with autoimmunity have lower amounts of *Lactobacillus* and *Bifidus*, and so recommends taking a broad based probiotic to restore these bacteria to your gut; as well as eating prebiotic foods. Thyroid hormones also have a large impact on glucose metabolism, and weight gain; and an underactive thyroid is linked to insulin resistance; and so it will also be linked, by implication, to **obesity** and **type 2 diabetes**.

Probiotics and Obesity, Coeliac Disease and Diabetes

Evidence linking changes in the gut microbiome to obesity, coeliac disease, and diabetes have begun to emerge recently, showing that probiotics positively affect the composition and/or function of the commensal microbiome and alter your immune responses.

Other studies showed that probiotics may reduce **body fat** and **weight gain**. (The strains used were Lactobacillus gasseri SBT 2055, Lactobacillus rhamnosus ATCC 53103, and the combination of L. rhamnosus ATCC 53102 and Bifidobacterium lactis Bb12).

One consistent factor in obesity is chronic inflammation, and this is borne out by examining the fat cells (adipose tissue) of obese individuals, which secrete inflammatory cytokines, whereas the fat cells in lean individuals have regulatory T cells that are anti-inflammatory, and so prevent inflammation.

Anti-obesity effects of anti-inflammatory probiotics has also been found in *Lactobacillus brevis* OK56 from a kimchi lactic acid bacteria collection, which is an example of how prebiotics are also beneficial to health (Kimchi is a fermented food).

Probiotics and Inflammatory Bowel Disease – Crohn's Disease and Ulcerative colitis

The two main inflammatory bowel diseases are **Crohn's disease** and **Ulcerative Colitis**, with both having chronic inflammation of the intestinal tract. Studies show that patients with these disorders have a deficiency of *Firmicutes* (for example Lactobacillus) and *Bacteroidetes* (for example Bacteroides). (Similar names unfortunately!).

The studies also show that **Crohn's Disease** is actually a series of disease states and that some forms may be treated by reversing this imbalance in the gut microbiome.

Other studies show that *Bacteroides fragilis* protects animals from **Colitis** that has been caused by *Helicobacter hepaticus.*

Probiotics have also been shown to directly reduce gut inflammation in people with constipation, although the numbers in this trial were small.

Probiotics and disorders outside of the Gut

The leap, from believing that probiotics can treat gut related disorders, to probiotics possibly preventing or reversing other chronic disorders has taken some considerable time. However, recent studies now show that probiotics, by returning the gut microbiome to homeostasis (balance), keep the gut lining (the epithelium) healthy, helping to protect it against gut permeability (leaky gut) among other things, including providing fuel for our body (like butyrate), and making neurotransmitters and vitamins.

We also read earlier that probiotics also impact the immune system in the gut, which, in turn, protects you from chronic disorders. I will explain the impact of probiotics on specific chronic disorders below, although this is not intended to be a full explanation of the disorder (each of which would need their own book!)

Probiotics and cravings

I am repeating what I wrote in the chapter on the gut-brain connection, but I include it here for completeness, as I think it may be helpful.

There have been few studies to research gut permeability in alcohol dependent humans, but one study observed a decrease in *Bifidobacterium* and *Lactobacillus* in the stool cultures of alcohol dependent subjects with liver damage compared with those of healthy controls.

The microbiome of these people was restored with the probiotics ***Bifidobacterium bifidum*** and ***Lactobacillus plantarum 8PA3***, and patients with alcohol-induced liver injury showed a greater improvement after taking these probiotics, rather than standard therapy alone.

In addition to restoring the gut lining, other studies show that probiotics also have an effect on the immune system, reducing inflammation by producing anti-inflammatory cytokines, which may also help people with liver damage.

It seems possible that, as an imbalance in the gut microbiome can lead to cravings for alcohol in someone who is alcohol dependent, it may also cause **cravings** for **nicotine** in smokers after they have withdrawn from cigarettes for a few weeks. Not because of the nicotine, but because different gut bacteria influence behaviour, and

144

someone's behaviour when smoking may beneficially affect some bacteria (food choices could destroy the 'good' bacteria in your gut for example); and so some bacteria may prefer it if their host smokes cigarettes. This is just my opinion, but it seems to be at least possible.

People who want to stop smoking are often concerned about weight gain, and this may not be due to just eating more. Recent studies have shown that people who stop **smoking** have an increase of *Firmicutes* which help get the most nutrients from food and also store any excess as fat.Taking a probiotic to counter this should prevent such weight gain!

Probiotics and Allergic Diseases

It is difficult to demonstrate an exact effect of probiotics on **asthma, allergic rhinitis (hay fever),** and **food allergy**, as it is with many disorders, because of the limitations when studying humans (for example, the many different strains of gut bacteria which may affect the disorders, the duration of the study, only having a short follow-up period, and not being able to limit all other lifestyle and dietary factors which may also impact on the diseases.). However, many studies have demonstrated a *significant* clinical improvement in **atopic dermatitis** with the use of probiotics, and probiotics may also improve both the symptoms and the quality of life in patients with **allergic rhinitis (hay fever).**

Many studies are conflicting in their results regarding probiotics and asthma, but all the ones I read had very small sample sizes and really needed additional research to confirm their findings. However, one study found that a combination of *both* probiotics and prebiotics prevents **asthma-like symptoms** in infants with atopic dermatitis.

Other studies indicate that taking the probiotic *L. rhamnosus*, with minute traces of peanut protein, can stop **allergic reaction to peanuts**.

Probiotics and Metabolic Syndrome (also called Insulin Resistance Syndrome)

Metabolic syndrome is a combination of several conditions, consisting of increased blood pressure, high blood sugar levels, abdominal **obesity** and abnormal cholesterol levels. They increase your risk of **heart disease, stroke** and **diabetes**. Having just one of these conditions doesn't mean you have metabolic syndrome (insulin resistance syndrome).

Studies showing the effects of three different strains of probiotics (two *Lactobacillus* and one *Bifidobacterium*) given individually, on metabolic syndrome, in subjects on a high fat diet; suggested that probiotics which target the gut microbiome may prevent, or help reduce, **obesity** and those related metabolic conditions mentioned above.

(The strains, for those who would like to know, were *Lactobacillus paracasei CNCM I-4270 (LC), L. rhamnosus I-3690 (LR) and Bifidobacterium animalis subsp. lactis I-2494 (BA)*).

Probiotics and Anxiety, Autism, Depression, Dementia, Alzheimer's disease, Epilepsy and Schizophrenia

In addition to direct links between probiotics and health, there is increasing evidence to suggest that there is an interaction between the microbes (the microbiome) in the gut, and the central nervous system (CNS) in what is recognized as the microbiome–gut–brain axis. This impacts on disorders like **anxiety** and **depression**.

Much research is now happening to see if treatment with prebiotics, supplements, and probiotics are a viable strategy to treat several brain disorders, when used together with conventional medications. Some suggest that probiotics may be beneficial in preventing **Alzheimer's disease**, where protein deposits in the brain bind to glutamate receptors, which then prevent impulses from passing from one nerve to another (reducing memory functions for example). A solution to this may lie with the gut bacteria (which can be taken as a probiotic) which convert glutamate to GABA, a calming neurotransmitter which prevents the action of these proteins in the brain. Early life **stress** in rodents can be reversed by the probiotic *Lactobacillus* which increases levels of both *Lactobacillus* and *Bifidobacteria* in the gut; and, although early life stress can lead to **depression** in adulthood, this **depression** can be reversed by the probiotic *Bifidobacterium infantis*; suggesting that probiotics are useful in the treatment of these disorders.

Although the numbers are small, one study, published in the British Journal of Nutrition in 2011, found that a 30-day course of probiotic bacteria (a mix of *Lactobacillus helveticus* and *Bifidobacteria longum*) led to decreased **anxiety** and **depression** in healthy human volunteers.

Accumulating data in humans has been supported by a mouse model of **autism**, where behavioural abnormalities, impaired intestinal barrier function (leaky gut), and an altered microbiome can be helped by taking *Bacteroides fragilis*. Another way that leaky gut is linked to **anxiety** is that nerve-immune interaction can influence the mucus layer protecting the intestinal lining. As your gut microbiome controls these nerve-immune interactions in the gut, probiotics may also contribute towards healing leaky gut and reducing **anxiety** in this way too.

There have also been suggestions that toxins from 'bad' bacteria in the gut (or an overabundance of 'bad' microbes) can lead to brain changes such as **Alzheimer's disease** and **dementia**. Probiotics to restore the gut microbiome to balance may protect against this.

Gut bacteria, and humans, both produce amyloids, a type of protein, which is found in the brain of people suffering with many degenerative conditions, including **Alzheimer's disease**. Although there is no current research investigating this link, it may be possible that bacterial amyloids, if leaked into the body via leaky gut, could initiate deposits in the brain, interfering with normal brain function.

Taking a probiotic with large numbers of *lactobacillus* and *bifidobacteria* may improve **memory**, improve **brain disorders** and help **problem-solving**. Eating prebiotics (nutrients for gut bacteria) and taking a broad based probiotic may also lower the likelihood of brain seizures, thereby benefiting people with **epilepsy.**

Probiotics and Social Anxiety

Although it is now well established that taking probiotics, and also eating foods which nourish the gut microbiome, can alleviate **anxiety** and **depression**, little has been known about whether our gut microbiome can alleviate social anxiety or not. Until now. Recent studies showed that eating fermented foods like raw sauerkraut and kimchi, which naturally contain probiotics, reduces **social anxiety**. So, feeling **'shy'** or **awkward** in company may only be due to a dysbiosis in the gut microbiome (which can be changed by eating fermented foods and/or taking a broad based probiotic) rather than a fixed personality trait. Exciting news is that these fermented food probiotics also have a protective effect against **social anxiety** symptoms for those with the genes that make them more susceptible to being **socially anxious**. In other words those with a higher genetic risk; but there are environmental solutions to this risk.

An example of strains that are useful in reducing every day **anxiety** are *Lactobacillus acidophilus* Rosell–52 and *Bifidobacterium longum* Rosell-71, which are found in the Optibac 'For Every Day' probiotic.

Probiotics and gut health

Prescription drugs given to people to reduce inflammation of their joints, seen in some chronic disorders like **rheumatoid arthritis**, include non-steroidal anti-inflammatory drugs (**NSAIDs**); such as ibuprofen, diclofenac and indomethacin. NSAIDs also damage the lining of the stomach and intestines. The damage to the intestines can be prevented, and reduced, by the lactic acid produced by *Lactobacillus*, which are found naturally in your gut, but which may be taken as a probiotic if your gut bacteria are out of balance. Although many strains of *Lactobacillus* produce lactic acid, the strain used in a probiotic in one study was *Lactobacillus casei*.

Probiotics and your immune system, including general health

We read earlier in the book ('The link between all chronic and autoimmune disorders', chapter eight) that all chronic disorders are associated with chronic inflammation; and that chronic inflammation is caused by your immune system reacting to some trigger or triggers (see the chapter on the immune system earlier). We now know that some commensal bacteria, which are found in some probiotics, can alter this immune response; and the research into the different strains of gut bacteria is growing. Some bacterial strains that are known to date, that can modify immune responses, and reduce chronic inflammation, are *Lactobacillus rhamnosus*, *Lactobacillus reuteri* (strain 6475), and *Lactobacillus acidophilus*. The actual compounds that gut bacteria make, which have an effect on our body, are largely unknown at this time, but one that we do know is lactic acid, produced by *Lactobacillus*, and lactic acid is known to modulate our immune system.

One example of this can be seen in a study which showed that taking the probiotic *L. rhamnosus* significantly reduces the risk of getting **upper respiratory infections** in children.

Probiotics and Cardiovascular Disease

Although our circulatory system is exposed to risk factors, such as high blood pressure, cigarette smoking, or eating a diet high in sugary or fatty foods; the lining of our blood vessels protect us from hardening of the arteries, or blood clots, by making nitric oxide.

However, studies published in 2015 revealed that *Lactobacillus* in your gut microbiome also produces nitric oxide as a bi-product of digestion of food. **Nitric oxide** can modulate the immune system, and also has antibiotic properties.

Probiotics, Chronic Disorders and Aging

Our gut microbes decrease in number and diversity as we age, and this reduced microbiome is linked to many chronic disorders. It may explain why we associate many chronic disorders with older age; but taking probiotics to reverse this decline in our microbiome may also reverse our susceptibility to many chronic disorders. In other words, these chronic disorders are not *age* related but *microbiome* related, and the microbiome can be restored in days! Of course, if we do not feed our gut microbiome with the vegetables and soluble fibre it needs, it will not remain healthy!

Breaking news

The Office of Naval Research are sponsoring The Brain-Body Institute, Ontario, Canada; as researchers at the Institute think that a dysbiosis of intestinal bacteria caused by stressful situations, dietary changes, loss of sleep and living in submarines, may contribute significantly towards PTSD (post-traumatic stress disorder); but that treating people with antibiotics and then probiotics, to restore their diversity in their microbiome, could cure the PTSD, and also anxiety and depression. (Source: sciencedaily.com; Office of Naval Research; April 25, 2016).

Take home message for probiotics

Why eating/taking probiotics regularly can be helpful:

- They are natural antibiotics, and so kill of harmful bacteria and yeast.
- They make B vitamins and vitamin K.
- They protect against cancer and other disorders.

- They protect your gut lining and so help reverse conditions like Crohn's disease.
- They prevent skin problems, especially acne and eczema.
- They reduce blood levels of 'bad' cholesterol.
- They fight stress and food cravings, preventing or reversing anxiety, type 2 diabetes, obesity, and others.
- Many produce lactic acid, which aids food digestion.
- They are a factor in the prevention and reversal of chronic and autoimmune disorders; including **eczema, psoriasis, ulcerative colitis, Crohn's Disease, irritable bowel syndrome, cancers, food and other allergies, thyroiditis, type 2 diabetes, multiple sclerosis, obesity, rheumatoid arthritis** and many more.

Probiotic Sources

Coconut kefir, and fermented foods like sauerkraut and kimchi are good sources of probiotics. Many other vegetables can be cultured in the same way as kimchee; and you can make your own.

If you want to supplement your diet with a probiotic capsule; choose a brand that is pharmaceutical grade, with at least three different strains of friendly bacteria and between 5 to 20 billion live organisms.

Finally

Some possible good news is that large pharmaceutical companies are now heavily investing into researching the microbiome and the potential of probiotics. This will speed up the research into finding particular strains and should be helpful. My only concern is that they may then become very expensive, or only available on prescription. We need to ensure that our health comes before the profits of large companies and so remain vigilant!

Antibiotics and their impact on your 'good' bacteria

You will be familiar with the usefulness of antibiotics, and how they can save lives, but what most of us don't consider is that they kill off bacteria other than the ones they are targeting. In other words, they can also kill off your good bacteria. Some other prescription drugs can also affect your microbiome; but your bacteria react differently to different drugs!

Your gut bacteria, as we read earlier, can degrade drugs and remove them from your body. They can also change an inactive form of a drug into an active form that your body can then use. What wasn't known until recently is that all of these drugs, including antibiotics, may change the ongoing function of your bacteria.

For example, taking prescription drugs can result in your bacteria significantly increasing the expression of their genes that are involved in xenobiotic (drug) metabolism and degradation; while antibiotics induce expression of genes involved in vitamin production.

With continuing research, on how the gut microbiota directly and indirectly affects drug metabolism, more information is beginning to emerge.

Antibiotics may be useful if you have a small intestinal bacterial overgrowth however (SIBO), and also to treat other bacterial infections which may be life threatening if left untreated. Antibiotics cannot kill viruses however, and so we should take them only when necessary, if we want to have a healthy balanced microbiome.

Faecal Transplants to restore your gut microbiome to health

Faecal transplants are transplants of gut microbes from a healthy person to one suffering from a chronic disorder. At the time of writing, the only disorder that is treated by faecal transplants is that caused by *Clostridium difficile* which can colonise the gut after prolonged use of broad spectrum antibiotics (which kills off your good bacteria). *C. diff* produces toxins which damage the intestinal lining, leading to severe diarrhoea and colitis (inflammation of the colon), and can be life threatening (which is why medicine is more open to trying a novel treatment). Only people with recurrent infections of *C. diff* are considered for treatment. These infections can recur after antibiotic treatment, but are cured 83 to 100 per cent of the time after a faecal transplant.

There is only one company, called 'Openbiome', who supply the faecal transplant material, and they, of course, undergo rigorous safety testing.

The surprise to most people is that the faecal transplant treatment for this notoriously difficult-to-treat disorder had around a 90% success rate as, in medical terms, this level of success, using conventional medical treatments, for any disorder, is unheard of. Almost a miracle cure! On a BBC one programme in 2015 called Trust Me I'm A Doctor, one doctor who witnessed the treatment of a patient in the USA said, that if the doctor there trained her, she would use it on her patients without question on her return to England, as she was so impressed with the results.

I am hopeful that other disorders may be treated in a similar way in the future, but we read earlier that transplants are not always beneficial to the receiver. For example, transplants from obese mice to lean mice resulted in the lean mice becoming obese. Those experiments were to show that the different bacteria in the gut microbiome was implicated in obesity, but it hi-lights the fact that transplant material needs to be considered very carefully before the treatment becomes mainstream. Of course other effects can be seen that are beneficial, and some people treated may no longer suffer from depression for example. The point is that it needs to be regulated. In the meantime, taking a broad based probiotic and eating for a healthy microbiome will be a good start.

Dietary changes – You are what you Eat, Digest and Absorb

Let me start by saying that we are all unique, and so there cannot be one 'right' 'diet' for everyone. There are so many 'recommended' 'diets' out there that it really isn't surprising that most of us become very confused. What is 'healthy' after all?! I am going to answer this very simply, and I will start with that very word, 'healthy'. What, when applied to food and drinks, does it even mean? Health means the absence of disease, and so when we read that a particular food is 'healthy' we presume that it will protect us from disease, but one thing alone (often called a 'superfood) cannot keep us free from disease on its own, and so how can we redefine it? Simple. The food and drinks that we consume need to be **'nutritious'**! Your body needs **nutrients**, delivered in a way that humans have evolved to recognise, over hundreds of years, to use, to maintain a **healthy body, healthy weight, healthy mind** and **healthy wellbeing**. We can now look at foods and drinks that are *nutritious*. The ones that will give your body the nutrients it needs to function, and to protect it from diseases and **cancer**. Yes, that's right, if you give your body what it needs to eat, your body is amazing at fighting disease, repairing itself and even killing off cancer cells. I'm not saying that your body's systems will never go wrong, but give it the tools it needs and it is better than most prescription drugs at healing itself (and we can also get amazing help from our doctors if our body is struggling with acute diseases). However, take away the triggers which make it struggle and you have a fighting chance of staying well! So what are nutritious foods and drinks?

Your body has evolved to use proteins, carbohydrates, starches, vitamins and minerals from food (we also read that some of the food we eat, soluble fibre, is consumed by our gut bacteria which then provide us with some of the essential vitamins that we need to survive). A (basic) summary of the nutrients in different food categories can be found at the back of the book in the appendices, but I will give you a really easy plan to follow.

Your food plan

- Eat whole foods. In other words, the food that can be found in nature; like vegetables, fruits, rice, quinoa, wild fish and organic meat. I didn't include anything made with wheat flour, as the gluten in wheat flour, as well as causing disorders like coeliac disease, can cause leaky gut, and gluten sensitivity. Other flours are also for occasional use only.
- Eat 20ml of cold olive oil a day to protect against heart disease. Don't cook with it as this removes the benefits (laboratory results seen on Trust Me I'm a Doctor).
- As a guide, have approximately half of your plate covered with vegetables (you can include a little fruit for sweetness if you like to), a quarter with starchy carbohydrate like root vegetables, sweet potatoes or potatoes (root vegetables and sweet potatoes are not absorbed so quickly so keep your blood sugar more level), include a source of soluble fibre like beans, and, if you like meat and fish, add a small amount of one of these a couple of times a week (palm size, one centimetre thick as a rough guide). An alternative to meat can be soy products, but take care as the soy crop is now mainly genetically modified, and soy is also a known allergen.
Remember to eat a variety of different fruits and vegetables, as each one has a unique set of phytonutrients for you. Try adding a different one each week.
- You can get all of your protein from vegetables and from nuts and seeds, and so don't be afraid that you will be deficient in protein if you don't eat animal produce. However, different vegetables have different parts of

proteins that we need, and so you need to eat a good supply and variety of vegetables in your diet to get all the essential amino acids your body needs. The good news is that a pile of vegetables is filling but hasn't got as many calories as a pile of potatoes or a large chunk of meat!! If you choose to eat meat or fish, these are also a source of protein.

• Good fats. Eat nuts in moderation, as, although the fats they contain are good for us, too many will pile on the pounds! Another good source of fats is avocado. Our body needs fats, to make things like hormones, so they should not be excluded from our meals.

A typical **western diet** isn't very similar to this! In fact, meals often contain high fat, low amounts of soluble and insoluble fibre, added processed sugar and manufactured salt (rather than sea salt which also contains minerals). This type of food isn't just poor in nutrition for us, but it is also poor in nutrition for our 'good' gut microbes! If you struggle to make a complete change, try adding some fermented foods like raw sauerkraut to one meal a day, as this contains probiotics and also nutrients for your gut microbes. It is slightly sour and so will help retrain your taste away from sweet.

For meal tips, I have included some ideas in chapter nineteen, but think '**Mediterranean diet**' when you are looking for meal ideas and you won't go far wrong!!

For people who are concerned about their **weight**, what you eat affects the balance of *Firmicutes* (which promote weight gain) and *Bacteroidetes* (which are associated with being slim); and the secret lies mainly with fruit and vegetables! The polyphenols in fruit and vegetables not only boost *Bacteroidetes* but they inhibit *Firmicutes*. So, eating things like apples, blueberries, and grapes could help with weight loss; although a diet that includes a variety of different coloured fruits and vegetables is the optimal. Other things to help are drinking green tea, eating fermented foods (raw sauerkraut or kimchi) and also wine vinegars.

There is now strong evidence of the potential of prebiotics to afford protection against a range of chronic disorders common in humans, including **colorectal cancer, ischaemic heart disease, type 2 diabetes** and **obesity**.

As well as avoiding bread and other products made with wheat flour, as they can cause chronic disorders, you may notice that I haven't mentioned milk, yoghurt, cheese, or anything made from dairy. There are three reasons. The first is that we don't need it, and can get all of the nutrients we need, like **calcium**, from other sources like vegetables. For example, broccoli is a much better source of calcium than milk! The second is that it is also a trigger for some chronic disorders (see below!). The third (and this is an ethical rather than a health reason, and so not all will share my view) is because milk is needed by baby cows; and they are taken away from their mothers so that we can take the milk. After two or three pregnancies the mother is killed. Baby boy cows are also killed. Not great, especially when we don't even need it!

Dietary changes also include finding and avoiding food triggers of chronic disorders. This deserves its own section, which follows, and so let us look first of all at potential *food* triggers and then move on to *non-food* triggers. There is a twenty three day **elimination diet** for you to follow later in the book; so that you can find your own unique food triggers.

Breaking news!

- Some exciting new research into diet and health published November 2015, involving eight hundred people, showed that many factors are involved in chronic disorders which are not related to the actual content of the meal itself. For example, many other factors, including what we ate for previous meals, how long it was since we slept, how long it was since we exercised or are about to exercise, and the diversity and content of your gut microbiome.

- As the microbiome aspect of this research particularly interested me, it was exciting to see that the study found that some microbiomes are 'beneficial' in terms of chronic disorders associated with chronically impaired glucose control, like **type two diabetes, obesity, non-alcoholic fatty liver disease** and **coronary heart disease**; and these gut microbes, together with a change in diet and lifestyle, also reduce risk factors such as **HbA1c%** and **cholesterol** levels. The research was conducted in Israel and is ongoing, but it found that the results compared to studies of people in both the USA and Europe.

Take home message for prebiotics – dietary changes

- What you eat can change your gut microbiome in only a few days. Eating a good variety of vegetables, some fruits, and some protein (either nuts, seeds, tofu, quinoa and other vegetable sources, or a little organic meat or wild fish) will feed your 'good' health-giving bacteria, while starving out the bad bugs. Easy and nutritious solution to long term health!
- Occasionally, for most of us, going 'off-piste' will not do you any long term harm (unless you have a disorder like coeliac disease of course); but remember that you will have changed your gut microbiome into one that makes you unhealthy. However, it can revert to health with care so enjoy the party! Whatever you do, do not get stressed about it afterwards!

Avoid Triggers of Chronic disorders

This comprises food triggers and non-food triggers. We will start with food triggers.

Food Triggers

People have become very confused about 'advice' regarding which foods are good or bad for us; which seemingly changes from one year to the next. As I said at the beginning of this book, I have looked at the science behind this and I am passing on this science to you, in an unbiased manner, without any agenda. I don't want to get viewers to a TV programme or magazine, nor sell supplements or indeed sell the foods themselves. I have no agenda, other than to pass on information so that people can make informed decisions about their own health. Even selling this book is not my primary purpose, as I only wanted to write the book to inform you, so that you could help yourselves to achieve a healthy body and healthy mind. If this book can help just one person, then I have done my job.

The reason that people have become confused is because people in different camps are often advocating their own personal approach, sometimes driven by ego or by pre-determined biases. In addition, some media headlines are sensational in order to get viewers and sell stories; and so the results of some poor research is passed on to the public as fact. Thirdly, and probably the most important, is that humans are fixated with reducing things down to that one cause or one solution, and tend to take their eye off the bigger picture; the whole body. Once we look at our body as a whole, we see that no one *single* food is a 'superfood', and that we *all* need the same thing. The solution is easy – we need a variety and plentiful supply of different coloured vegetables, some fruit, and either nuts and seeds or a small amount of organic meat and wild fish. That is highly simplified, but you get the picture. Real food is the answer, and variety is key in order to get the full array of nutrients that you need.

My aim, when I took my degree, was always to use my knowledge to inform people and make their lives better. For this reason, and to cut through the confusion, I decided to undertake an unbiased review, of the masses of scientific literature, with tons of evidence, and see where it took me. The result was this book.

Let us continue now with food triggers. These are some of the most common, but if removing those does not help that doesn't mean that you do not have a food trigger, but that you haven't yet found it! Some fruits, some things like aspirin, and even the foods you eat routinely, may have a detrimental effect on your body. The best way to test this is to do an elimination diet, which is included later in the book, but, as we just said, these are the most common and so it might be helpful to start with these.

- **Processed foods including Processed Sugar**
- **Dairy**
- **Gluten from wheat, rye and barley**
- **I also add genetically modified foods to this list, which are still under debate, but I will explain my reasons for concern.**

Some foods are triggers because they either provoke an allergic response or you may be sensitive to them. You can find which of those foods do this by taking an elimination diet (in the chapter on **Elimination Diets**). As with many things that evolved over the last fifty years or so, our bodies have not adapted to recognise some things that are now widely accepted as 'food' and so don't respond to some foods as normal 'food'. These are processed foods.

Processed foods

Why processed foods confuse our digestive system

Processed foods, by definition, are not whole foods. In other words, you couldn't pick them from a tree or dig them up out of the ground as they don't exist in nature. The reason why these processed foods may confuse your digestive system is because our bodies have evolved over thousands of years to digest and absorb the whole foods that can be found naturally. We simply don't recognise these new processed 'foods' as food. The processed foods have been manufactured, or extracted or have additives of some kind; and some tins, bottles and packets list ingredients which look more like a chemistry lesson than a list of food ingredients. Some ingredients, like aspartame, can also be neurotoxic, and cause an increase in **epileptic seizures**.

If your body does not recognise the ingredients as food they will either eliminate them from your body, or may store them as toxins in either your fat cells or your joints, depending on whether your body considers them to be toxic or not.

Tests for safety of these ingredients are often done by examining one ingredient at a time, but we also know that, as we all have choices, we may eat combinations of many different additives at any one time. It isn't the fault of the producer, as they have tested the ingredients to the standards required of them, but they may be one of your triggers for your chronic disorder. Eliminating processed foods could therefore be a good start on your path towards a healthy body, healthy weight and healthy mind. Remember that 'new' foods like 'gluten-free' and 'vegan' which are marketed as 'healthy' alternatives are still processed foods. Fresh food is always best. Sorry!

One of these commonly eaten processed foods is sugar, which many of us will consider to be 'natural' as it is glucose. However, it has been extracted from the whole plant (sugar cane or sugar beet) and so sugar, unless it is inside a plant or fruit, is a processed food, and it is also able to fool your body.

But how can processed sugar confuse our body, when it is, after all, just glucose, which our body get from fruits, vegetables and grains, and uses all the time? Let us look at processed sugar in more detail.

Sugar

The confusion arises because your body does not know that you have managed to avoid the digestive process and miraculously arrive at one of the end products of digestion, glucose, without actually eating the equivalent amount of sugar beets or sugar cane. In other words, your body reacts the same as if you have just eaten vast quantities of the whole food in isolation from it, without all the associated fibre, vitamins, minerals, carbohydrate and fibre that it normally comes with. In fact, as it has bi-passed the digestion process altogether, and arrives in pure nutrient-only form, it can be, and is, rapidly absorbed into the bloodstream from the small intestines.

This creates a rapid rise in blood sugar levels, (you become *hyper*glycaemic, temporarily) which causes a rapid rise in insulin levels to bring blood sugar levels back down to normal levels. This is because too much glucose in the body, at any one time, is toxic to cells and body processes. It is positively harmful. If we continually eat sugar, or drink sugary drinks, and cause these rapid surges of insulin, the system can become fatigued and stop working properly, which in turn can lead to disorders like **diabetes** and **obesity**.

[*I should say here that although the return to normal levels will happen eventually, a surge of insulin into your bloodstream after eating sugar, causes your blood sugar levels to actually fall below normal levels first. You become hypoglycaemic (temporarily) before levels return to normal. It is this drop in blood sugar that can make you feel jittery, hungry, and in need of more sugar!*]

If sugar is so toxic though, why do we want to eat it? Surely our body will tell us when we have had enough? Well the reason we like sugar is that we are programmed to like sweet foods, like fruit, as they are a great source of quickly available energy for us. Children particularly like sweet foods. However, in nature, fruit is only available for a limited time in a particular geographical area and so before recent technology we would not have had the readily available 'all year' supplies that we now find in our supermarkets,; and so a desire for sugar wouldn't have been a problem. We couldn't eat it in excess as it was not available to us.

But even the year round availability of fruit isn't the real problem. The problem lies only with the fact that our digestive system simply hasn't evolved at the same rate as the food changes that we have seen over the last fifty years. Our body has evolved to give us 'full' signals when we have eaten enough, but as we haven't eaten the whole food these signals are bypassed. Too much sugar will make you feel sick of course, but you can eat an awful lot of sugar before that kicks in!

In people with normal blood sugar levels, insulin brings the blood glucose back to within a normal range by converting some of the glucose to glycogen, and storing it (mainly) in the liver (as we read in the chapter on digestion). Insulin also triggers your body to store fat, and so eating sugar can lead to weight gain and **obesity**, not just because of the calories you eat in a day (although of course that does matter), but because of *what* you eat; in this case, sugar.

The reason why sugar is particularly harmful to **pre-diabetic** people is that *continually* high blood sugar levels (**hyperglycaemia**) can cause **loss of sight, loss of limbs, heart problems** and **nerve damage**.

One of the reasons that blood glucose *remains* high is because you may have genes which make you susceptible to it (and this is the case for people from some parts of Asia). However, **the good news is that changes in diet and lifestyle can lower constantly high**

blood glucose levels even if you do have those genes which make you susceptible to it.

When you have an excess of glucose (glyco-) in the blood it binds to haemoglobin (Hb), the protein in red blood cells that carries oxygen throughout your body; and the haemoglobin becomes *glyco*sylated or glycated. The test for glycated haemoglobin, which is also a test for diabetes, is **HbA1c**, which needs to be at a level recommended by your doctor.

Breaking news

- Studies published in January 2016 show that a pregnant mother who is both **obese** and has **diabetes**, increases the risk of **autism** in her child.
- Although the *reasons* for this have not yet been established, as the relationship between the gut and the brain is a more recent area of research; I would suggest that the root causes of both the diabetes and the obesity, which we are finding solutions for in this book, also contribute towards chronic disorders in the brain as well as other parts of the body. This gut-brain connection is also being found in other brain disorders like **Alzheimer's disease, epilepsy, multiple sclerosis** and **attention deficit disorder**. We read about this connection in the chapter on the gut-brain connection.

Sugar substitutes - Breaking news!

- In 2014 it was found that some sugar substitutes, like saccharin, also affect the bacteria in your gut; and that these changes in your microbiome induce glucose intolerance.

Additives - Breaking news!

- According to research published in Nature on 25th February 2015, artificial preservatives used in many processed foods could increase the risk of **inflammatory bowel diseases** and

metabolic disorders. Some chemicals, called emulsifiers, which are widely used (even in products considered to be 'healthy' alternatives) were found to alter the bacteria in the colon. This is the first time that additives have been shown to affect health directly.

Dairy products (i.e. from cow's milk)

The reason why cow's milk has been used for infant formula, and as a food, after weaning, is because it has a similarity to human milk. However, as cows have been bred for various favourable characteristics over the years, their milk, which used to be something called A2, is now A1. Sufferers of asthma may be advised to avoid dairy, or try alternative milk products like goats milk, which is an A2 milk, however, both A1 and A2 milks are associated with human disorders.

For example, recent European investigations have shown a reduction in **autistic** and **schizophrenic** symptoms after decreasing A1 milk intake. The study also showed that the root cause of both of these disorders is very similar; with both reacting adversely to dairy and wheat products. Animal trials have also supported the linking of **type-1 diabetes** to milk exposure in general, and A1 beta-casein in particular.

In spite of this, cow's milk and dairy products are recommended by most Western societies because they are a source of calcium and protein. However, in 2009, it was shown, for the first time, that milk promotes *most* chronic diseases of Western societies; including **coronary heart disease, diabetes mellitus, cancer, hypertension, obesity, dementia,** and **allergic diseases**.

A long term study published in 2003, investigating research over a 20-year period; also confirmed that A1 cow's milk is significantly and positively correlated with **ischaemic heart disease**, in 20 affluent countries.

165

Dairy proteins are similar to gluten; and so if you are sensitive to dairy products, you are also likely to be sensitive to other things that it is cross-reactive with, like gluten; and so eating either will provoke an immune response once it has been triggered.

Dairy may also cause things which seem totally unrelated to digestion. For example, Dr Izabella Wentz found that her **acid reflux** and **carpel tunnel syndrome** both disappeared after removing dairy from her diet. (*Reversing Hashimoto's, webinar, 24 March 2016; Dr Izabella Wentz*). You can read more about this, and **Hashimoto's thyroiditis**, on her website, *Thyroid Pharmacist*.

There are now some great alternatives to animal milk, and so our choices are expanding. They include oat milk and almond milks. (There are also soy milks but this can be genetically modified unless it is organic, and soy is also a known allergen and so should be consumed with that in mind). So, as a reminder:

- Intensive dairy cattle breeding may have emphasised a genetic variant in milk (A1), which has adverse effects in humans.
- Oat milk and almond milk are two non-dairy alternatives to milk.

An interesting fact about consuming dairy products is that we are only able to do so if we have the genetic mutation which allows us to digest lactose, a protein found in cow's milk. This mutation results in us still producing the enzyme lactase, which breaks down the lactose in order for us to be able to digest and absorb it. We hear about 'lactose intolerance' as though this is a problem, when in actual fact, those of us that can digest cow's milk have 'lactase persistence'. In other words, we are still making an enzyme that normally stops being produced in our body after weaning (although we are able to still produce it as children for a while).

The mutation is thought to have occurred in populations that started to farm dairy cows and eat dairy products. People who had this mutation, in times of poor nutrition availability, would have thrived much better than people without the mutation, and so this mutation was passed down through generations. It is not abnormal for adults to be unable to digest milk though. We are not meant to drink milk as we have been weaned onto solid foods!

Gluten (from wheat, rye and barley)

People are often confused when they hear about gluten being bad for us, but we have discussed earlier in the book, in chapter nine, with the timeline, how gluten can indeed cause health problems. The good news is that not all gluten *is* bad for us! There is gluten in other foods, like oats, rice and quinoa, but the problems lie with the particular gluten in wheat, rye and barley, and possibly the main culprit may be wheat gluten. Why so? I must admit that when I started to read the research I came to it with a very sceptical mind, as humans have been eating bread for years. However, the tests to detect coeliac disease are fairly recent, and ones for gluten sensitivity are only being researched now! The problem may therefore have been an inability to diagnose, rather than a recent problem with gluten.

One possible explanation of why gluten in food affects those of us who do not suffer from coeliac disease (but have non-coeliac gluten sensitivity) is that coeliac-triggering gluten proteins are produced at higher levels in modern cereals. In addition, these new strains of modern wheat, which are high-yielding, have been used for human foods without animal or human safety testing. We also read, in the section on dairy products, that wheat and dairy are cross-reactive, and both are now known to be linked to many chronic disorders.

A useful website for those with coeliac disease in the UK can be found at the coeliac disease charity website, with some useful information on diet and lifestyle to be found here: https://www.coeliac.org.uk/gluten-free-diet-and-lifestyle/gf-diet/gluten/. It gives advice on where gluten can be found and the risks involved. For example, it does say that although gluten can be found in some lipsticks, the amount is not likely to cause problems; but I think it is useful to know about these things.

Another useful website may be that of Dr Isabella Wentz, who studies **Hashimoto's thyroiditis**, and who suggests that both gluten and dairy (including goat's milk) can trigger this autoimmune disease.

Studies to differentiate between **coeliac disease** and **non-coeliac gluten sensitivity (NCGS)** suggest that exposure to environmental factors, including wheat, for a prolonged period of time, may result in **inflammatory bowel disease** or **Crohn's disease**. NCGS can also result in many autoimmune conditions, including **Type 1 diabetes, arthritis, thyroiditis,** and even 'brain' conditions, such as **multiple sclerosis.**

Most people with coeliac disease will recover when eating a gluten-free diet; but a small percentage do not. When this was investigated it was discovered that milk could also provoke an immune reaction, similar to that against wheat. Some other foods tested (oats, coffee yeast, corn, oats, millet and rice) although seeming to provoke an immune response, only did so because they had been contaminated with gluten. However, if your gluten free diet does not result in a return to health, it may be useful to use an elimination diet to try avoiding the above foods.

- *The following foods were found to be safe for coeliac disease and gluten-sensitive individuals: sesame, buckwheat, sorghum, hemp, amaranth, quinoa and tapioca.*

If you have any symptoms of any chronic disorder, like those listed in the introduction to this book, it may be beneficial to avoid gluten. A good way to try this is with the elimination diet in chapter fifteen.

Genetically Modified Foods

The herbicide Roundup®, of which glyphosate is the active ingredient, is the most widely used herbicide, and it is sprayed on GM crops for both humans and animals, and on some non-GM crops, to ripen them or prior to harvest (for example it is sprayed on non-organic wheat before harvest).

Glyphosate is found in some foods, like non-organic bread, and it reduces the number of your 'good bacteria' (*Lactobacillus* and *Bifidobacterium*), but it does not harm pathogenic bacteria like *Salmonella* and *Clostridium* species, which are highly resistant to glyphosate.

A reduction of beneficial bacteria in the gut microbiome by ingestion of glyphosate could, therefore, disturb your normal gut bacterial community. In other words, it could cause a dysbiosis, an imbalance, in your microbiome, with associated links to chronic disorders. It may be that, in some cases, non-gluten sensitivity may be caused not by the gluten *per se* but by the herbicide that was sprayed on it before harvest.

Some studies suggest that glyphosate is linked to pineal gland dysfunction, which, in turn, is associated with many neurological disorders including **autism, depression, dementia, anxiety disorder** and **Parkinson's disease**.

Studies into the accepted industry standard period of testing (three months) imply that longer-term (two year) feeding trials need to be conducted to thoroughly evaluate the safety of GM foods and pesticides in the formulations used commercially.

Alcohol

I include alcohol here because it causes leaky gut, but it is only temporary and stops as soon as the alcohol has left your system.

Avoid non-food triggers for chronic disorders

We have already discussed food as being a possible trigger of chronic disorders, and what **we eat certainly plays the major part**, but there are also *other* triggers in our environment that can contribute towards chronic disorders, so how do we know what is safe?

Safe or not safe?

The fact that some substances used in our environment and in our foods are now banned (for example DDT, a pesticide which was made by Monsanto, and some artificial food colours are no longer used); shows that a lack of available research at any particular time does not necessarily mean that something is safe or OK to use or eat. Why does this happen though? Surely things are tested for safety before we use them or eat them aren't they?

Well, for many years, authorities around the world have developed a 'safe until proven otherwise' approach to new substances, with little or possibly ineffective research *proving* their safety before use by the general public. For example, studies to determine the safety of some additives may focus only on that one additive, and not on the effects that it may have when combined with other things; or the tests may only happen for a few months and so long term effects are not seen. It is another example of 'micro-science', focusing on the 'one result', much as I mentioned earlier in the book relating to medicine and how we treat only one part of the body, looking at one 'system' in isolation and treating those particular symptoms. To be fair, in many ways it would be almost impossible to look at every possible combination, and it would be excessively expensive to do so, but my point is that this research relies on us living with, or eating, only one (potentially harmful) thing at a time. Who lives like that? Who eats like that? No-one. In addition, most of these things have evolved over a very short time period, with many being introduced in only the last fifty years. Lots of new things for your body to respond to. They may be outside of your control, but before you panic, there is a solution! Read on!

What we *can* do – things that *are* in our control

We can't protect ourselves from every single manufactured chemical introduced to us in our products and in some of the food we eat, but that is only if we continue to use them and eat them of course.

We may not be able to change policies of governments or business but we *can* change our own environment and our own home. As more of us do this, then that will have an impact on our greater environment as profits lead change for big business and this will also impact on government decisions; firstly because they need the taxes from business to provide services, and secondly because they want to help their constituents and so will try their best to act on their behalf.

So what are these triggers? They can be found in all sorts of things including:

- Air pollutants – for example from vehicle exhaust
- Cosmetics – some ingredients
- Household products – some ingredients
- Pollen
- Paint (low VOC paints are available. Lakeland for example)
- Food additives
- Altered 'food' like trans-fats and emulsifiers
- Shampoos
- Products for the face and body

- Products for laundry
- Air pollution – air 'fresheners' in the home (can change, once in the air, to toxic substances like formaldehyde)
- Pesticides/herbicides (eat organic to avoid these)
- Heavy metals (like aluminium)
- Table salt (use sea salt, as this has added minerals)

There are many things that can cause us problems, and being 'natural' isn't necessarily the solution as Aloe Vera can irritate some skins. Sodium lauryl sulphate (SLS) is the product that creates a lather in soap and shampoo, but it can dry the skin. It is even used in some body lotions, and on the TV programme 'Trust me I'm a Doctor' with Dr Michael Mosely, I was surprised to learn that it is even included in some creams for eczema, a condition of excessively dry skin! Many people are avoiding SLS now, but we need to make sure that the alternative we choose is a healthy one, in that it is suitable for our own body. As I said earlier, we are unique and some will be affected more than others, and so we need to have our own personal plan, which we can only really find by trying and eliminating, as products on the shelves are all classed as fine for us to use. As I mentioned earlier, this classification isn't necessarily a reassurance of complete safety, and tests to prove this would be too expensive.

I'm not going to be prescriptive here and suggest particular things to use (I share with you what I personally use in the appendices at the end of this book), but would recommend trying different things and seeing how your hair/skin/body respond to them. If your hair is stronger and naturally shinier without having to add another chemical to make it so then the product is working! As each of us is different we can also react differently to each product. However, anything that isn't healthy is out of balance, so don't accept things like 'dry skin' as the norm!

As for air pollution, then clearly we can't control the entire external air that we breathe, but there are some simple steps that we can take, even in a busy city. For example, planting trees to the front of the house, or putting plants in pots on a balcony, will protect us from some external vehicle pollution as the plants kindly detox the air for us. Some plants are recommended as good air detoxifiers, and a chat with your local garden centre will give you all the information you need to buy the right plants for your particular needs and location.

Another solution when out walking is to walk as far away from the road as possible. Even a few feet can make a difference to the amount of air pollution that we breathe. Of course using eco-friendly transport and electric cars without exhaust fumes would also help to reduce air pollution too.

Take home message

- You can't control what other people do, including businesses and governments, but you can choose what products you use and what food you eat; and so you can change your personal environment, and that of your home.
- There are healthy products in the market, often found by people selling organic products, or at health food stores. The people who work at those stores often have researched the products that they sell and so can help you with your choices.
- The main thing to remember is that you are in control, and the second thing to remember is not to get stressed about anything that isn't under your control, because stress can be bad for us!!! I mention why in the next section of solutions.

Right, you have now restored your gut microbiome to a healthy balanced state, and you are feeding those bacteria in order to keep yourself healthy and joyful, and you are avoiding triggers. Fantastic!!

Well done you amazing person!! You have conquered Everest, so well done! ☺

You are nearly there, but there are two other things you need to be careful with, and those are stress and sleep.

Please remember that although we can't always avoid some of the potential triggers, the main thing to do is not to worry about it, as stress can contribute, in a major way, towards getting chronic disorders!! Lack of sleep can also impact on your health. I will explain more in this chapter, but bear in mind that you *can* achieve a healthy body, healthy weight, healthy mind, and healthy wellbeing, and this book will help you to achieve exactly that.

Stress

So what *is* stress? Well *some* stress is good for you and helps you in times of danger (fight or flight response) but many of us have low level *continual* stress and that isn't good for us at all! What do I mean by low level stress? I mean worrying about tomorrow, being annoyed about what happened yesterday, and any thought which take you out of the present moment. I'm not going to talk too much about this in my book, other than to say that there are some great books on the subject (living in the now); but I am going to talk about what happens in your body when you have those stressful thoughts, and how this can lead to ill health.

When you have a stressful thought, your brain reacts in the same way as if you are in danger and also that the event is happening right now. In other words, if you are feeling angry about what someone said yesterday, you feel your stress levels rise, and your body reacts in exactly the same way as if you were being chased by a tiger. Right now. Every time you re-think it, the same reaction in your body occurs. It is like the event happening over and over again. Each time, your brain receives a 'danger' (stress) thought and this triggers the fight or flight response. But what does this response involve?

174

Well, your thoughts of danger trigger a release of hormones by your brain, which then cause your adrenal glands to release (extra) cortisol into your bloodstream. I say 'extra' because you have cortisol in your blood all the time, as it is necessary for many things, including regulating your blood sugar levels and your metabolism; but in times of danger (or stress), extra cortisol is released by your adrenal glands to help you deal with the situation. In other words, this extra cortisol causes you to release adrenaline, which causes a release of extra glucose into your blood and muscles, giving you the energy to fight or run.

However, as I mentioned at the beginning of this section, most of us don't need to run away from a tiger or even to fight anything; we just have continual low level stress, and so what stresses or dangers are causing your extra release of cortisol and what effects does it have?

I said that the initial trigger, in the brain, was from 'thoughts' of danger (or stress). As we said, the brain does not know whether these thoughts are triggered from a tiger approaching or from being stuck in traffic or annoyed at what your boss said yesterday. The response is the same. Your thoughts, about *perceived* stress, create production of a stress hormone, cortisol. However, in addition to cortisol you also produce adrenaline, and, if you do not run or fight, this can make you feel anxious as your heart rate increases. If you don't run or fight, insulin then reduces the excess glucose out of your blood, which can (temporarily) make you hypoglycaemic (blood sugar is below normal levels) which in turn can make you feel jittery and crave sugar! The adrenal glands can also become over-worked which can leave you feeling exhausted, or wired, or both.

Cortisol also stays in the bloodstream for a while, as it aims to replenish the glucose it released to enable you to run from the tiger. It replaces your body's energy stores. How? By making you hungry. So 'thought' about being stuck in traffic, or what your boss said, can increase your appetite and also lead to **obesity** if prolonged!

*[TIP: **If I feel stressed, I actually pump my arms rapidly in a running action for about fifteen seconds. This releases tension and stops any stress. I think it must fool my body into thinking than I am really running!! Actually, it probably burns off some of the excess sugar!**].*

To summarise, thoughts, about the future and the past, can make your body feel the same as if it is under attack and needs to protect itself from danger. Don't be too concerned though, as there are very easy ways to gain back control of your mind, and decide which thoughts you want to follow! There are some great books and online videos to watch, as well as some great tips on relaxation for your body and mind, and I will reference these at the end of the book in '**further reading**' for those who are interested.

However, one other aspect of this 'fight or flight' response, which is triggered by your thoughts, is that **it also affects your digestive system**. The link may not be too obvious at first, but once we realise that the last thing your body needs to be concentrating on, while being chased by a tiger, is digestion of your food, it makes more sense. In times of danger (or perceived danger by your brain in response to stressful thoughts) your body wants to concentrate energy into your muscles (cortisol releases stored glucose to give extra energy to your muscles) and increase your heart rate (adrenaline does this) which pumps blood faster in order to get this extra energy into your muscles so that you can run or fight. **It also temporarily shuts down your digestive system.** This, in times of being chased by a tiger, would not be a problem, but if you are worrying constantly about things in the past or things that may happen in the future, it isn't difficult to see how this can impact on your digestive system in the long term.

Breaking news!

- Recent research into the way the mind works, by the psychiatrist Judson Brewer, shows that we have a hardwired system in our brain to learn about the things that help us to survive. It is the 'trigger – action – reward' system. For example:

  • You are hungry and you find a food that is tasty (trigger),

  • You eat it (action) and

  • It makes you feel good (reward).

Your brain remembers this food as something that makes you feel good, but, as well as applying it to a food needed for survival, it also applies that memory to other situations. For example, if you feel anxious your brain remembers that thing that made you feel good, in this case a particular food, and sends a strong craving for it, so that you will feel good instead of anxious. In other words, the trigger, instead of being hunger, is stress, and the action is to eat the food which your brain has already established makes you feel good... Because the reward for eating that particular food (feeling good) is already hardwired into your brain, you stop feeling stressed (temporarily).

Part of our brain does actually try to tell us not to do things which are harmful to our body, but this area (the pre-frontal cortex) shuts down if we are stressed and we revert to old habits, our default from previously learned behaviour. The difficulty we have if we try to force ourselves not to respond in this way is that the process is hardwired into our 'survival' part of the brain, and this is why it is so difficult to stop.

However, there is a solution!! Instead of fighting the impulse to eat cake, smoke a cigarette or drink alcohol, Judson Brewer (psychiatrist) found that if you become curious about what you want, rather than following emotions of 'wanting' blindly, you aren't dragged into the part of the brain that 'craves' something; to the part of the brain that remembers that the food made you feel good. Simply by being consciously aware, the 'cravings' part of your brain quietens down. But why does that happen?

Well, your brain enjoys being curious, it finds it rewarding (so there is the 'reward' part of the trigger – action – reward response), By being curiously aware of all of your senses when you eat the food, drink alcohol, or smoke a cigarette, your mind loses interest in them as a 'reward', as the curiosity is reward enough. In other words, although the trigger (stressful one) is still there, and the memory to eat/drink/smoke to make you feel good remains, your mind loses interest in it as a reward because it has another reward. Presumably the curious awareness is a more interesting reward than the food/drink/cigarette.

Judson Brewer (judsonbrewer.com) has two apps available, one for food cravings is coming out in 2016 and the one for stopping smoking is http://www.cravingtoquit.com; but he says that the same curious awareness would also apply to things like 'having' to check your twitter feed or Facebook constantly.

Take home message:

- Low level stress results in extra cortisol (which can increase appetite and may lead to obesity), and adrenaline (which may cause anxiety and chronic fatigue or being wired or both) and also a supressed digestive system. BUT! By being curious, you can change the 'trigger-response-reward' response from a stress/anxiety producing one to a curious aware one. By simply being curious (which your brain finds 'rewarding'), the part of your mind that becomes activated during low level stress responses actually quietens down! You can also apply this conscious awareness to any compulsive thought, like 'having' to respond to texts, or 'wanting' a cigarette, or a 'need' to check your twitter feed. For further information, there are now apps available, by Dr Judson Brewer; two of which are mentioned above.

Are there any other links between stress and our digestive system? Yes there are, and stress may be linked to the food that you eat, and so let us look at that now.

Stress and food

We mentioned in the section on your microbiome that some bacteria can make neurotransmitters like serotonin, the happy hormone, and other microbes, which produce toxins, can make you feel bad; and so we know that having a healthy balanced microbiome, by eating healthy whole foods and avoiding harmful triggers, can also lead to a healthy mind and feelings of wellbeing. Eating healthy whole foods, with lots of plants, can therefore impact on your stress levels, as they can make happy hormones which also helps with stress levels.

Some studies suggest that eating a high protein diet, long term, can reduce short-term, but not long-term, memory and also impair the ability to cope with acute stress.

Cortisol, as well as being a stress hormone, is also involved in food digestion and metabolism; and so eating more in the morning, while cortisol levels are at their highest, and less in the evening, when cortisol levels are low, results in less fat deposits in the body. Eating the same foods, but at different times (later in the day) results in more fat being deposited in your body than if you ate those same foods earlier in the day. (Source: 'Trust me I'm a Doctor', Michael Mosely, live experiment and lab results; November 2015).

Stress and the *way* you eat

The way you eat can also impact on your health and on your stress levels. When you eat quickly, or eat at your desk, or watch television, you aren't actually concentrating on the food, but on the taste and maybe the heat/cold of the food (or maybe the television!). While the sensation of eating is important to the enjoyment of food it mainly satisfies your mind and not your body. To see what I mean try this. The next time you eat, make a conscious effort to relax your body, lower your shoulders, and breathe more slowly. Then be aware of the actual food, and chewing it. Slowly appreciate it. This will make you feel relaxed and you will be much more in tune with what your body actually needs, rather than overruling thoughts that shout about what your mind fancies.

Of course the speed you eat also affects your body's ability to get the feedback message to you that you are full. If you eat quickly it hasn't got time!! But how does this link to stress? Well, by changing the way you eat, being aware of the food and eating in a more relaxed manner, this also reduces stress. Why? As you eat quickly, with a sense of urgency (maybe we think we haven't got 'time' or need to 'hurry' to get our work done), then this 'thought', as we just mentioned, also impacts on your stress responses. Your body reacts as it would to any other stressful situation, releasing cortisol, which in turn impacts on your digestion. So, just before you eat your first mouthful, take a slow breath in and out and relax any tension in your shoulders. Then focus on the food and enjoy!

Stress, your immune system and your whole body response

We already mentioned that stress temporarily suppresses your digestive system, but it also turns down your immune responses and also impacts all other endocrine responses like thyroid hormones. In other words, your whole body is affected. Your body does this because in a time of perceived 'danger' or 'alarm' it needs all of its resources to deal with the 'threat' to your life. Of course there isn't such a threat, but your body doesn't know that.

Thoughts can also override your 'full' signals, but why do we want to? Obviously we are all aware that eating too much will pile on the weight, but why do we do it? Why do we eat more than our body needs? Well the reasons are similar to those of what happens when we eat quickly, in that we aren't actually consciously thinking about the food at all, but listening only to thoughts of 'wanting' which can override all the body's signals, evolved over years, which tell us that we are full or that we don't really need something. Being aware, slowing down and eating consciously (rather than grazing while watching TV or having your mind elsewhere), will open you to being aware of your body's signals and not just your mind's signals. Eating slowly, and chewing your food also releases digestive enzymes which break down the food so that you can digest and absorb it.

Stress and your microbiome

Your mind can 'want' things because of neurotransmitters produced by particular microbes, and we read earlier that there is an established link between the gut and the brain, and so don't worry too much about 'willpower', as changing your gut microbiome can also change your old bad habits! To summarise, eating foods to feed your microbiome can help you reduce stress levels and potentially reduce cravings.

As with all lifestyle changes that we talk about in this book, probiotics can be useful. In this case for example, enhancing your microbiome by taking probiotics such as ***Lactobacillus rhamnosus*** can be useful in the treatment of anxiety caused by raised cortisol levels. We talk much more about this in the section on probiotics.

Finally, remember that ghrelin, the hunger hormone, is also produced in response to inflammation in your gut. If you heal your gut, by taking probiotics, eating vegetables and avoiding triggers, you may then produce less ghrelin and feel less hungry.

Stress and exercise

A third lifestyle change you can make is to take some exercise. We all know that we should, but most of us don't really know what happens if we don't. It doesn't have to involve a gym unless you want it to. Walking, dance classes, swimming, and any physical movement all count. If you need motivation, think about taking a dog for a walk (borrow one if you haven't got one!). It is well documented that a lack of exercise impacts badly on your joints (they seize up like any machine that isn't used!), mental health (exercise released endorphins, which make you feel great), and sleep patterns (we all sleep better when we do some exercise).

If you exercise outside, by walking for example, you gain an extra benefit from daylight, as this enables your body to make vitamin D. It also impacts directly on your brain, improving your wellbeing.

Stress and daylight

If we do our exercise outside then this incorporates the fourth thing we need which is daylight! The exercise can be as simple as walking, and we don't have to jog to keep ourselves fit, but a gentle stroll probably won't burn off many calories! A brisk walk (you can build up to this) or walking up some hills or inclines will do the trick!

As we just said, daylight causes your body to make vitamin D, which is necessary for healthy bones, but it is also necessary for health and the prevention of many chronic disorders.

Daylight is also important in setting your 'body clock' which determines your **sleep patterns**. It also improves mental health, as nature has a calming effect, quietening thoughts. It also sends signals directly through your eyes straight to your hippocampus in your brain, and **the happy hormone serotonin is produced**! However, daylight in winter may not be enough to produce sufficient serotonin, and this is why some people suffer with seasonal adjustment disorder

(SAD). This can easily be resolved by buying a SAD lamp, and it doesn't have to be expensive. I bought the mini SAD daylight lamp and we all love it. It feels like the sun is shining into the room and it really lifts your spirits. It is best to only have it on early in the day, because if you use it at night you may not feel sleepy. Vitamin D is also known to alleviate low mood associated with dark winter months, and you can take this either from some foods, like salmon and eggs, or by taking a supplement. Long term vitamin D3 supplement seems to be more effective at keeping body levels up in the winter months, compared to vitamin D2.

The dots are joining. Already we can see the link between thoughts, stress, food, exercise, daylight, sleep, and potential chronic disorders; as well as ways to prevent and reverse these. Let us look a little more about **remedies** for one of the biggest culprits of stress, and that is stressful thoughts.

Stress and meditation – You don't need to sit cross-legged or have closed eyes for this

Simple meditation can just be taking a few (mindful) breaths. Slow breaths, concentrating only on your breathing. A good way to stop your mind chatter interfering (taking your attention away to thoughts it is making), is to ask yourself the question 'am I still breathing?' **For that brief moment, your mind is quiet. That is meditation.** An example I like to give is to be more like a dog! Be aware. What can you see, hear, feel, and smell? That is what life is like for a dog. They don't let their mind drag them off into (often useless) thoughts; but are present here, in the present moment, in the now. That is why we love being with them. We sense that they are present.

You may have read that stress is 'just' a thought. Most of us react badly to that suggestion as it feels so urgent and important to us, but unless you are genuinely in some danger and need to fight or run, then maybe you might want to consider your thought responses to situations (which in turn cause you to feel stress). I have made these changes myself (over a couple of years) and now am amazed at how many years I believed that those thoughts *were* me rather than just part of me. I now know that I don't have to react. If your situation needs to change, then thoughts that plan those changes are good ones; but thinking fearful thoughts about your situation is not helpful and will add to your stress.

There are many books which can help, but two books by Eckhart Tolle were particularly helpful to me and these are 'The Power of Now' and 'A New Earth: Create a Better Life'.

Another amazing book is by Ken Verni Psy.D., and it is called 'Practical Mindfulness. A step-by-step guide'. As the name suggests the latter one offers practical help, and has some great tips, such as how to unravel stress, how to deal with change, and how to achieve good communication. It also includes three week meditation programmes to follow too if you want them.

There are many videos available online which offer suggestions of different types of relaxation exercise or meditation exercise. The thing that I liked is that they do not ask that you *follow* any teachings, and they don't affect any religious beliefs that you hold, but, for me, in relation to stress, most of what they say can be summarised into a simple realisation, and that is:

Stress (and worry) arises because of the gap between 'what is', in other words the present situation, and what the mind 'wants' it to be. For example, if the mind 'wants' it to be sunny on a rainy day, and complains, and you follow those thoughts, then you will feel a degree of stress because it isn't sunny. However, if you accept that it isn't sunny, and don't have thoughts about dissatisfaction, then no stress arises! The main realisation for me was that however much I may 'want' it to be sunny, or complain that it isn't sunny, it isn't going to change the situation. It isn't going to make it sunny! In other words, the stress, or pain, from the thoughts, created by the mind, which want the situation to be different from what it is, are an additional *layer* on top of 'what is' and that layer is stress. I was amazed to find that the difference in my thoughts towards a situation did, and does, actually change things. My only suggestion would be to try it and see. I don't ask that you believe or disbelieve what I am saying, just try it for yourself if you want to.

As we said earlier, another helpful practice is some meditation; not necessarily what you may think of as meditation, but maybe just taking time outside in a green space, or going for a walk, or doing yoga, or art. In other words, anything which makes you feel joyful.

I'm not a spiritual teacher and so will leave that to the experts, but what I can tell you is that life can be joyful. Challenges will always come, but the way that you then deal with those challenges determines whether you will feel stressed or not.

Meditation for busy people

Kris Carr has an amazing album that you can buy online, called 'Meditation for busy people'. There are ten, and each one lasts for four to twelve minutes. Two of them are specifically for when you wake up and before you go to sleep; and they make me feel so tranquil, relaxed, and blissfully content! For more details, go to her website http://kriscarr.com/products/self-care-for-busy-people-digital-meditation-album/. Meditation, or mindfulness, as a daily habit, can change your life.

Breaking news!!

The science that explains mindfulness and 'ego'.

Recent research into the way our brains work has revealed that we have two areas of the brain that are involved in thought. One area is active when we are retrieving thoughts from the past or making plans for the future, a sort of internal thought process which is our **default**

mode network (DMN) (the posterior cingulate cortex to be precise!); and the other is active when we are dealing with the present moment, and is the **pre-frontal cortex (PFC)**.

If you have read any books at all about mindfulness this will be ringing bells, as many refer to the 'ego' as being the source of constant mind chatter, involved only with past or future and always dragging us way from the present moment. They refer to it as the 'egoic' part of the brain because it relates to 'self' (ego means self). It doesn't get good press, as moving away from the present moment and being dominated by the 'egoic' mind is also associated with fearful thoughts, anxiety, dissatisfaction and a lifetime of never ending wanting!

The thought that we have a selfish demanding 'egoic' bit of brain, that we have to overcome, is not a nice thought, especially if we then see others as being dominated by this alleged 'self-centred' and rather unpleasant stream of thinking; but that was how it seemed to be. **Until now.**

The thing that puzzled me is that we are social beings and so why would we evolve to be self-serving, as this doesn't work well in relationships at all! I began to join the dots. Was there something happening in our brain that could explain this? The answer is YES!

I looked at what was happening in our brain when we are anxious, and wondered if there was an alternative view of our 'egoic' mind. It seemed to me that the way our default mode network (DMN) works could give it a scientific context; but if we recognise that our DMN is merely a source of stored memories, raised as thoughts, which suggest things to help alleviate a discomfort of some kind, based on its memory bank of the tried and tested; then the thoughts coming from that part of the brain can be recognised as ones intended to be helpful, and there for survival, rather than to be purely selfish and unpleasant. They are also suggestions, and not directions, and so it is possible to override them and I will explain how shortly.

I also suspect that that the reason so many people are having problems with constant 'mind chatter', which they are looking to calm down with 'mindfulness' techniques, is because our environment has changed drastically over the last sixty years. We are constantly bombarded with sensory stimulation of many kinds, which triggers a response from our DMN, as it constantly tries to warn us of something or find a solution for us, especially after hearing and reading constant bad news and alarming media stories. The result? A constant internal stream of thoughts, suggestions, 'mind-chatter'. To know how to change this, I needed to know more about how it worked.

So how does the 'default mode' work? Well it is the area of the brain that remembers things that are necessary for our survival and wellbeing; for example, find a sweet food like fruit, eat it, it makes you feel good, so remember what the food is and where to find it for another time. The same applies to warning us of danger. The process of learning and storing the memory is one of trigger (feel hungry) – action (find the fruit and eat it) – reward (hunger gone, feel good) – repeat, and these memories are stored in our default mode network (DMN). However, our creative brain uses this information for things other than remembering to eat healthy food like fruits, because many of the 'chemicals' we eat, smoke and drink actually hijack the *same* brain pathways as the ones that make us feel 'good'. They hijack our 'survival' pathways to make us want them. So a cigarette or a sugary cake triggers our default network to remember them as necessary for our *survival*, and each time we smoke a cigarette or eat a cake we reinforce the 'habit loop'. So, the good news is that you don't have a part of your brain that is selfish, or on 'self-destruct', it is trying to help, but the bad news is that our lifestyle can hijack it. This will make sense to many of us, who 'know' that what we eat or drink isn't good for us but do it anyway as it is difficult not to.

The reason it is so difficult is because in addition to it trying to help, the DMN is also *very* resistant to being ignored. Survival is a pretty strong instinct right! So when you have tried the smoking/drinking/eating and rooted the 'trigger-action-reward' in your default brain, it stays there; and we all know how difficult it is to resist that cigarette or glass of wine, no matter how much we want to. Your default brain thinks it is necessary for your survival, so it is not going to let you stop easily! 'Self-control' or 'willpower' invariably fails, so can we stop the cycle? The answer is YES!

Dr Justin Brewer, psychiatrist and cravings expert, has worked on this subject for many years and has found that the solution lies in finding an alternative 'reward' (remember the 'trigger-action-reward-repeat' process employed by your default brain). The way to do this is simple but effective, and it doesn't meet with resistance, like willpower does. *The solution? Curiosity. Dr Brewer has found that our brain finds curiosity hugely rewarding!* That makes sense, as curiosity finds solutions. So how does it work?

Dr Brewer looked at MRI images of brains when they were having cravings, and found that our default mode network was activated, as it tried to come up with a solution to feelings of hunger/nicotine withdrawal and so on. However, by being **actively curious**, focusing on sensations of what is happening 'right now', being *aware* of the *sensations* in your body, the default mode network *stopped* being active. Although the curiosity didn't *remove* the craving memory, say for a cigarette, the default mode network lost interest in it and stopped being active; which meant that **the craving also stopped**. In other words, our default brain stopped searching for a memory to help, because a different part of our brain, that was curious about the present moment, was establishing a new trigger-action-reward-repeat pattern to help us, and to be stored as default.

Your pre-frontal cortex, the part of your brain which deals with the present moment, the 'now', seems to override the default mode network, which is only involved in past or future. Your pre-frontal cortex is also the part of your brain that 'knows' that you shouldn't eat the fourth biscuit and that smoking damages your health, but it is also the part of your brain which becomes fatigued and then goes offline when you are stressed, hungry, angry, lonely or tired, and so you revert to your default network for help! Don't despair, there is a solution.

This is where mindfulness or meditation techniques come into play, they are simple, they need only take a few minutes each time, and they work. You don't even have to like doing them, as just the act itself will work, and will establish new patterns of 'trigger-action-reward' in your brain. The reason they work is because they calm the default mode network, because we are focusing on the present moment rather than past or present, and you are creating a new, alternative reward (curiosity, awareness, of the present moment) which your brain seems to prefer. It isn't easy at first because it is new to us, and will not bring an end to cravings overnight, but it *is* possible, and with practice it becomes easier and easier. You will gradually notice a shift, and may even feel a resistance to a lack of desire for a biscuit or a cigarette as memories of feeling good surface (remember that they are false memories, and are only there because your brain has been hijacked); but keep going, as once the new thoughts become an established pattern in your default mode network you will feel both physically and mentally better.

Essentially, the scientists are saying the same thing as many spiritual teachers, in that being fully aware of 'the now', rather than be dragged into our DMN, calms thoughts, which are intended to be helpful for survival but, because of sensory overload and constant low level stress, are often negative and fearful. Once the default mode is calmed, and we do not need its helpful suggestions (at that moment), it leaves us feeling connected with the present moment, being aware of our senses and feeling the joy of that. Joy, we realise, comes from inside, rather than from external factors; and joy, it seems is our intended default. That isn't the same as 'happiness', which is fleeting, but a deep sense of joy that remains throughout all of life's challenges, which will always be there; a cushion of resilience for future challenges.

Dr Brewer and his team have developed an app to help people stop smoking, and there will be an app for eating addiction later in 2016. For more information you can visit his website, http://www.judsonbrewer.com/

Take home message

- Eating for your microbiome keeps your neurotransmitters and hormones in balance.
- Eating quickly causes cortisol release in response to a stress trigger, which then impacts on digestion of your food
- Stressful thoughts trigger stress hormones like cortisol and adrenaline; which shut down other body responses, including digestion and your immune system.
- Exercise prevents joints from 'seizing up' and also releases feel good endorphins. Exercise outside (walking is fine) also produces vitamin D3 in your body, triggers production of serotonin (happy hormone) triggers production of melatonin (sets sleep pattern) and sets your body clock (so that you are in line with daylight hours).
- Being in line with daylight hours also brings you into line with your cortisol levels, which are at their highest in the morning and gradually deplete during the day. Cortisol as well as being a stress hormone, is also involved in food digestion and metabolism; and so eating more in the morning, while cortisol levels are high, and less in the

evening, when cortisol levels are low, results in less fat deposits in the body (Source: 'Trust me I'm a Doctor', Michael Mosely, live experiment and lab results; November 2015).

- Meditation can mean a walk in the fresh air or a couple of deep slow mindful breaths. Finding a meditation, or mindfulness routine, that suits you, brings your brain's logical frontal cortex into play, which dominates and calms your brain's default mode network (I call it our software), which is the source of 'mind chatter' (sometimes negative and fearful, as it is trying to keep you safe, and warn you of impending 'doom' as it sees it. In our busy world, this 'doom' very rarely exists, and so the thoughts, your software, need to be up-dated with a new 'app'!).

- New thoughts, created by mindfulness and your frontal cortex, create new 'software' in your default mode network, which you can then draw on for future experiences in life. In other words, you are creating a new piece of software, which also happens to make life more joyful and much less stressful.

Finally, another factor which can impact on your health is sleep, or rather a lack of it!

Sleep

Most of us know that we need a reasonable amount of sleep to function well, but what happens if we don't? For example, most of us don't realise that all of the waste products in the brain, like **dead cells and excess neurotransmitters** that haven't been needed and are floating freely, **are removed during sleep**; and that this is **essential for the health of your brain**.

When we talked about stress and cortisol I said that you have cortisol in your blood all the time, but it is at its highest in the morning when you wake. However, when sleep patterns are disrupted then cortisol levels can also be disrupted, and, as we read earlier, this can result in increased appetite and weight gain, as well as anxiety. It is well known that lack of sleep can lead to many neurological effects and a reduction in wellbeing.

There are some simple steps which aid a restful sleep and these include:

- Not looking at a 'screen' before sleeping (laptop, mobile phone, iPad and so on) as these emit a light similar to broad daylight, and fools your brain into thinking that it isn't time to sleep yet. In other words, it affects your 'body clock' as your brain is in harmony with light and dark and produces a hormone called melatonin which tells you to either be alert or to prepare for sleep. (As anyone with a small child will know, blackout curtains are necessary in summer to convince them that it really is time for bed!).
- Reducing lights and preparing your body to be ready for sleep, possibly by taking a warm bath or reading a book, together with having a fairly regular bedtime (10 or 11pm perhaps) gets you into the routine of regular sleeping times (but don't read your iPad in bed!)

In order to feel sleepy at the right time of day, it is important to go outside and get some daylight, as this sets your 'body clock'

Take home message

- Low level continual stress and lack of sleep can impact badly on your microbiome and on your health; but both can be brought back to normal levels, by diet and lifestyle, and you can feel better again.

The thing that amazed me most over the past year while I have been researching for this book, is how well chronic disorders respond to the health protocols we have been reading about in this book (probiotics, removal of triggers and so on). Disorders, labelled as progressive and untreatable, can be put into remission and even reversed in some cases, and that fills me with hope and gratitude. Hope, because we can help ourselves to become well, and gratitude for wonderful nourishing food that is also a 'medicine' for us. ('Remission' is different to 'cure', in medicine, because if we bring back the triggers the disorder can return, but if we keep away from the triggers we are effectively 'cured'. In other words, we have no symptoms, no antibodies, and no biological markers of a 'disease' (like HbA1c for type 2 diabetes). This can be seen in coeliac disease when people do not eat gluten.).

In other words, remove your trigger(s), manage stress and sleep levels, heal your gut, and you heal your body. That applies to all chronic disorders and allergies, unless the particular organ has been destroyed by antibodies, as can be seen in type 1 diabetes and some cases of underactive thyroid disorder. The result? A healthy body, healthy mind, healthy wellbeing. Even in those two disorders I just mentioned, you can prevent any *other* autoimmune conditions from starting (which is often seen) and may also reduce the need for as much medication for the disorder you have.

Well done you amazing person, you have nearly got through the whole book and now know how to make the changes that you need!! In addition to that, there are also some supplements which you may want to take, to help you on your journey, and some of these are listed below. If you do decide to take any of them, please make sure that the company that you buy them from uses organic or other ingredients which do not look like a chemistry lesson, and is of pharmaceutical grade! Also, and most importantly, always check with your doctor before taking supplements, in case they interact with medication that you are taking, or impact on any medical complaint that you have.

Chapter Fourteen

Supplements and Condiments

There are various supplements thought to heal the gut, maintain a healthy gut, alleviate mood swings, improve immunity, help eliminate *Candida albicans* abundance, and help restore a good balance of gut microbes. Before you take any supplements however, I advise you to talk with your doctor first, particularly if you are taking medication or have a health issue, in order to check that the supplement does not interact with your medication.

Berberine

Berberine has strong antifungal properties and has been shown to inhibit the growth of *Candida albicans*.

In addition, berberine has been shown to reduce blood glucose, and so may be a useful treatment for metabolic syndrome and the prevention of diabetes type two.

However, in some cases, Candida can be very persistent and many methods to reduce their number fail. In response to this the French have treated it with:

Saccromyces Boulardii,

This is also a yeast, but it does not adhere to your gut lining. It seems to prevent Candida albicans from adhering to the gut lining. Optibac sell capsules of Saccromyces Boulardii, which I did use for a limited time, and still do after parties and big feasts!

Garlic

Unfortunately there are no formal publications to back up anecdotal evidence regarding garlic and *Candida albicans*, but that doesn't mean it doesn't work, just that there aren't any studies! However, there are studies which show that garlic has anti-fungal properties, and many beneficial antioxidant and antimicrobial properties, one of which is that garlic is able to kill the most common bacteria which causes tummy upsets (*Campylobacter jejuni*); and it kills it more quickly and more effectively than antibiotics.

The ingredient in garlic which kills the bacteria is **diallyl disulphide**, which is released upon crushing the garlic.

Glutamine

Glutamine is an amino acid that is essential for many cell processes, and plays a vital part in the growth and maintenance of your healthy gut lining; protecting you from leaky gut. It also protects against oxidative stress (which is increased in autism spectrum disorders).

Your body makes glutamine from food supplies, and so rather than take a supplement, you can get it from food sources, such as raw spinach, grass fed meat, organic eggs, beans and leafy vegetables. However, in times of physical or emotional stress it may be beneficial to take a supplement, in the form of L-glutamine, as levels can become depleted in such circumstances. A supplement may be useful as we have been reading throughout this book about the importance of a healthy gut lining, as leaky gut leads to chronic disorders, but you should check with your doctor first, before taking any supplements.

Coconut oil

You can reduce a *Candida albicans* overabundance in your gut naturally, with a low sugar high plant food diet, but Candida makes you want to eat sugar and the cravings can be really strong! Eating a little coconut oil can prevent and end an overabundance of *Candida*, which I found diminished cravings for sweet foods and also alcohol. Of course you will then need to practice healthy habits, like reducing your sugar intake, decreasing stress, and eating a balanced diet full of vegetables. Also, other supplements, like berberine and *saccromyces boulardii* will help to get your *Candida* levels in balance again.

Candida overabundance causes symptoms that you may not associate with a fungal overgrowth; for example, sinus infections, blurred vision, foggy brain, moodiness, sugar cravings, and fatigue to name a few. You can see how it might be a natural reaction to just treat the symptoms of each of these individually and still not get to the root cause.

Oregano oil

One study shows that herbal therapy is as effective as antibiotics for treating small intestine bacterial overgrowth **(SIBO)**.

Liquorice

Liquorice contains glycyrrhizic acid, an anti-inflammatory, which is also effective in destroying and inhibiting **H. Pylori** and so is useful to treat and protect from peptic ulcers. When used in a gel, liquorice extract is also effective in treating **atopic dermatitis (eczema)**. Anecdotally, liquorice has helped people with low level anxiety and depression. As research evidence suggests that both of these conditions exist in a continuum, liquorice may be useful for people with sub-clinical symptoms; but care should be taken as liquorice is also linked to high blood pressure and so should be taken in moderation, if taking it at all, and always, as with any supplement, after discussion with your doctor.

St John's Wort

St John's Wort has been found to aid people with low level anxiety and depression.

Tryptophan

Tryptophan increases brain serotonin, and so may help us cope with stress. Although tryptophan can be found in foods, it is also available as a supplement.

Ginger

Ginger (*Zingiber officinale*) is used all over the world in cooking, and I prefer to use fresh ginger, but if you are not using it in your cooking it can also be bought as a supplement.

Ginger has been shown to prevent and **reduce cancer**, and is an **anti-inflammatory**, as it blocks the action of pro-inflammatory cytokines.

Turmeric

Turmeric is another spice and it is part of the ginger family and can be bought fresh from some fruit and vegetable shops, or online from Abel and Cole. It looks like a dark orange ginger rhizome, and has been used in Indian cultures traditionally to treat **asthma, heartburn, peptic ulcers, arthritis** and **wound healing.**

However, there is now evidence-based research which shows that turmeric, and its active constituent curcumin, is effective in treating a variety of disorders. Human clinical trials have demonstrated no toxic effects at doses of 1-8g /day / 6-8 months.

In addition to this, there is now clear evidence that curcumin (the active ingredient in turmeric) is therapeutic in many chronic disorders, including **Alzheimer's disease, Parkinson's disease, multiple sclerosis, epilepsy, cerebral injury, cardiovascular disease, cancer, allergy, asthma, bronchitis, colitis, rheumatoid arthritis, renal ischemia, psoriasis, diabetes, obesity, depression,** and **fatigue.**

As a comparison to traditional medication, curcumin was found to be as effective as seven different classifications of drugs, including **atorvastatin** (a statin, used in the treatment of diabetes type 2), **corticosteroids** (which are used in the treatment of allergies, skin conditions, ulcerative colitis, arthritis and breathing disorders), **fluoxetine** (an antidepressant), and **aspirin** (when used as a blood thinner). It also enhances the effectiveness of **oxaliplatin**, a drug used for **bowel cancer**. The protective and therapeutic effects of the curcumin in some (but not all) of these cases seems to be by a protection of endothelial and/or capillary barrier function. In other words, curcumin may protect against 'leaky' barriers.

Turmeric is not easily absorbed during digestion and so is said to have poor 'bioavailability'. In spite of this it is still effective as described above, but its bioavailability can be increased, and two ways to do this are by mixing it with a healthy fat, like olive oil, or with black pepper.

Chilli pepper, black pepper, liquorice, nutmeg and sage

These all have anti-inflammatory properties, even when just extracted from ground raw material and not used as concentrated extracts.

Vitamin C

People with high blood glucose levels are at risk of type 2 diabetes; and a measure of these blood glucose levels can be detected by measuring how much sugar has attached to the haemoglobin (Hb) in your blood (haemoglobin is your oxygen carrier). The test that doctors do looks at your HbA1c. High blood glucose levels results in high HbA1c. Vitamin C can reduce this HbA1c.

Vitamin B12

If you do not eat animal products you can be deficient in vitamin B12, although some vegetarian foods contain substantial amounts of vitamin B12. These include tempe (fermented soy), and some seaweed, including dried green laver (Enteromorpha sp.) and purple laver (Porphyra sp.). An example of quantity, is that 4 g of dried purple laver will give the daily recommended amount needed.

SIBO treatment

(Many natural medicine practitioners suggest that a combination of oregano, garlic, ginger, liquorice and berberine, among others, are useful for treating SIBO. I share this for your interest, although I could not find any research. However, that doesn't mean that it doesn't work, as research is expensive and needs to be funded).

I am not an expert on these supplements, and so if you are considering taking any, I would suggest that you take advice, both from your doctor (to make sure they don't react with any drugs that you are taking) and possibly a qualified herbalist. I decided to try them after listening to The Autoimmune Summit speakers, one of whom was **Dr Amy Myers MD**, who includes some of them in her book '**The Autoimmune solution**'; which you may want to read, as she specialises in the thyroid gland.

Vitamin D

You may have read that there are two types of vitamin D, vitamin D2 and vitamin D3. Vitamin D3 is the one that humans make, as a result of sunlight on their skin, and this is the vitamin that is also found in fish oil (which is sometimes used to make supplements). Both vitamin D2 and D3 are converted in the body and aid with our absorption of calcium (needed for strong bones and teeth).

In addition to being needed for healthy bones, vitamin D is necessary for many functions of the body, including our immune system; and this is why vitamin D deficiency can result in autoimmune diseases like type one diabetes.

Vitamin D3 seems to be better at maintaining levels of vitamin D in our body throughout the winter.

Olive oil

On 'Trust me I'm a Doctor' the labs showed that around twenty millilitres (two desert spoons) of (uncooked) olive oil a day helps to prevent **cardiovascular** problems. They tested proteins in urine, which can accurately *detect* changes in the disease itself, in real time, rather than merely *predict* it (for example by checking **cholesterol** levels). Any olive oil worked, it didn't need to be expensive, although there are now organic ones which, in my opinion, may be preferable, but not necessary. No other oil was found to have this protective effect. This may explain the benefits of the '**Mediterranean diet**'.

Milk thistle

If our intestines are not functioning optimally they do not remove toxins from our body as efficiently and so these pass in the blood stream to our liver; which can become congested. Milk thistle appears to help the liver detoxify, helping to reduce the symptoms of some chronic disorders; but it may react with some medications and disorders and you should always check with your doctor before taking it, as with all supplements.

Take home message:

- Some supplements may be useful, but I am merely sharing this information for your information and this is not intended in any way as a recommendation. You should always consult your medical practitioner before taking any supplement.

We need to find our triggers, and mainly the ones found in food as this is what comes into contact with our gut microbiome and intestinal immune system. How do you find your food triggers though? The elimination diet in the next chapter tells you how.

Chapter Fifteen

Elimination Diet

This is the gold standard to determine whether any foods or drinks are affecting your health. You remove all potentially harmful triggers, listed below, for twenty three days, and then re-introduce them, one at a time. You then see how you feel. If you feel energised, and vital, then the food you are eating is boosting the good bacteria in your gut, which are then producing the serotonin, happy hormone, and other vitamins and neurotransmitters essential for a healthy and happy life. If however, you've got brain fog, headaches, can't sleep well, or have other indications that things aren't optimal, then remove it from your diet, as it is triggering a potentially harmful reaction and may also be feeding the bad microbes in your gut. It may also be causing Leaky gut, which we know is a contributor to chronic and autoimmune disorders.

Lots of issues in this book are complex, and need explanations, but this one is simple. Heal your gut and you may heal yourself. Many of your disorders should improve; hopefully drastically (just as my asthma and susceptibility to colds have) and may actually disappear altogether (depending on the level of damage, if any, to your organs).

Although blood tests for sensitivity to foods are available, they can be expensive and they can also give false results. The gold standard for testing to see if you have a food sensitivity is by doing an elimination diet and observing yourself for changes in your body and mind.

Doing an elimination diet could give surprising results, as you may not even realise that you could feel a different way if you have always eaten your 'trigger'. That certainly happened with my mum, who told me that she now realised that she had suffered with low level anxiety all of her life. An elimination diet is a simple way to prevent a lifetime of inflammation, chronic disease symptoms, and even life-threatening diseases.

There are many examples of elimination diets, but some are very complicated to follow. This is an easy to follow, five step plan, which is useful to absolutely everyone, as we all want to prevent or reverse chronic disorders which can be brought about by food sensitivities.

The 23-day elimination diet – five easy steps

The reason why we do the elimination diet for twenty three days is because your immune system takes approximately twenty three days before the immune response to the trigger stops, and we start to feel the benefit of not eating that food. This elimination diet is simple, and has only five easy steps.

Step 1. Inventory

Before you begin your elimination diet, make a list of everything you notice in your body, no matter how subtle the symptom is, and no matter how long you have had it. Once you take this 'inventory', you will then be able to notice changes when they happen. Some of the more obvious symptoms with food sensitivities are shown below, but note down everything that you notice, even if it isn't included here.

Skin issues (like irritations and rashes)

Digestive issues (gas/bloating/diarrhoea/constipation)

Allergies (asthma, eczema, hay fever)

Low energy levels

Migraines

Seizures

Mood swings

Brain fog or other problems with concentration

Anxiety or depression

Acid reflux

Frequent colds, headaches and illness

Difficulty sleeping

Restless leg syndrome

Fibromyalgia

Thyroid problems (which can include feeling hotter, or colder, than those around you; and weight problems)

Symptoms of autoimmune disorders (such as coeliac disease, rheumatoid arthritis, multiple sclerosis and so on)

Weight gain or difficulty losing weight

Attention Deficit disorder or autism

Joint pain

If you suspect that your child has food sensitivities, they can have any of the above and may also have frequent bed wetting.

Step 2. Elimination

This elimination diet focuses on the main culprits. However, if you try this and do not feel better then it doesn't mean you don't have a trigger, but that you just haven't found it yet. Starting with the most obvious is a great start though! These are the six main culprits to take out of your diet. (It is only twenty three days!!)

No gluten (from wheat, barley and rye)*

No dairy (from cows, but also from other animals like goats and sheep)

No eggs

No soy

No processed food (ready meals with additives, processed sugar)

No nightshade family (potatoes, aubergines, tomatoes)

No alcohol

We include alcohol for several reasons. Firstly, it contributes towards Leaky Gut while you are drinking it, secondly, it has a lot of sugar that helps things like yeast and harmful bacteria in your gut thrive, thirdly it is a sleep disruptor and, last of all, it is a depressant. So when you eliminate alcohol, you may feel better in a few weeks, not just because of the absence of alcohol, but because you've actually changed your gut microbiome to one which keeps you healthy, and have removed some stress triggers from your life!

The nightshade family is included because they can be inflammatory and contribute to Leaky Gut, which is reversible when you stop eating them. They may not affect everyone but that is why we include them in your personalised elimination diet, as we are all unique!

If you are using this elimination diet with your child or children, please make sure to discuss it with your doctor or Health Visitor first, and they may also suggest useful tips. For example, my Health Visitor told me that broccoli was a brilliant source of calcium and a great alternative to dairy. However, a nurse also told me that a rash on my eldest son's tummy was nappy rash, which I knew could not be the case as he was never left in a wet nappy; and although I always advise working with health professionals, you know your child better than anyone; so I researched possible causes and eliminated eggs from his diet and the rash disappeared.

You can also make it a fun thing for the child to do, and also include them in the decision process so they don't feel deprived or resistant to changes. Once a child recognises the link between a food trigger and an adverse reaction in their body, they are both willing and empowered to make the right decisions for their health. For life. Although the nightshade family is included above, you may not want to eliminate potatoes from the diet of a growing child, as they need a good source of carbohydrates to provide the huge amount of energy they use! You could always try your child with sweet potatoes sometimes as an alternative if you wish to. As with any other suggestions above, please discuss this with your medical practitioner before making major changes.

My tip: If you are wondering what to eat if you don't eat potatoes, try parsnips. They cut up into chips and you can roast them in the oven with a little oil. They also mash well. You can do this with other root vegetables of your choice and they are all surprisingly filling! Experiment, and try mixing them together for different tastes.

*I should say here that you may want to see how your body reacts to organic bread as opposed to non-organic bread, as organic wheat has not been sprayed with glyphosate. As healthy bread is a good source of B vitamins, if we can find one that doesn't contribute to chronic disorders that would be wonderful!

Step 3. Make the changes

You can do this. It may take a few extra minutes a day to prepare food, and some changes in our weekly shop, but these are easy changes to make once you get used to them. New habits take 21 days to form, and so after twenty three days these new habits will be part of your (healthy) life! I have included some ideas for meals in chapter 21 to make life easier for you.

Step 4. Your shopping guide

This is also simple, as you eat whole foods that have not been processed, and do not come with a list of ingredients which look like a chemistry lesson. (It is preferable to eat organic foods where possible, as these do not have pesticides and herbicides which may also be a trigger for you).

Simply, these are:

Mainly vegetables, legumes (beans and lentils), seaweeds, and

Gluten-free grains like quinoa (unless you are not sensitive to gluten) together with

A small amount of protein, like nuts and seeds, or, if you want to eat animal produce, eat organic, free range, hormone-free meat or wild fish (that is low in mercury) plus

Healthy fats found in olive oil, coconut oil, sunflower oil, flax oil, walnut oil, and avocados. On 'Trust me I'm a Doctor' the labs showed that around twenty millilitres of (uncooked) olive oil a day helps to prevent **cardiovascular** problems. They tested proteins in urine, which can accurately *detect* changes in the disease itself, in real time, rather than merely predict it (for example by checking cholesterol levels). Any olive oil worked, it didn't need to be expensive, although there are now organic ones which, in my opinion, may be preferable (as they avoid pesticides), but not necessary. No other oil was found to have this protective effect. This may explain the benefits of the '**Mediterranean diet**'.

The fresh whole foods, and unprocessed meals you make yourself will have lots of soluble fibre, which will also feed your good bacteria which, in turn, will keep you healthy and happy. Also, the soluble fibre in vegetables and fruits make us feel full and control our weight.

If you like milk and cheese, then there are plant based alternatives, such as **almond milk** and '**Violife**' **cheese** (which is made from coconut oil and not soy). It is also possible to make your own 'milk' from nuts. **Pure** make a sunflower spread, as an alternative to butter, which they say does not contain emulsifiers; or you can find a healthy nutritious alternative of your choice.

If you do eat fish, try to avoid those with a high mercury content, like tuna and swordfish, as mercury is linked to some chronic disorders; and eat sustainably caught wild fish.

Organic free range meat is preferable for many reasons, including that it has not been pumped full of antibiotics, nor has it been fed with genetically modified soy (these 'extra' genes make products which have been found in goats milk, although in theory that should not happen).

If you do need an emergency breakfast bar, there are organic **Be'ond** bars or **Nak'd** bars, which are just cold pressed fruit and nuts. Nothing else added! **Nak'd** now also make 'salted caramel nibbles'. They taste like sweeties but are just 100% natural; with 96% fruit and nuts, and 4% rice flour and natural flavouring. Healthy snacking!

Although gluten-free breads, cereals and biscuits are available, they are still refined carbohydrates, with a ready supply of easily digested sugars; and so, in an ideal world, it is best to keep them to a minimum. However, in the short term, it can be a good way to help you remove gluten from your diet until you get used to making the changes in your meal plans.

I found a super easy, super-fast, no knead recipe on the pack of organic brown bread flour by Doves Farm. It is so delicious, and you can add seeds if you want to. All you have to do is put all the ingredients in a bowl and whisk. Leave in a bread tin until risen (you can leave it for hours!) and then bake for thirty minutes. There is also an even more simple organic bread mix available, by Amisa.

- *Please remember that newly arising foods like 'gluten-free', or 'vegan' processed foods and ready meals are still that. Processed. If you do eat them, have them very occasionally rather than include them in your meal plans for the week. Swapping one western style diet for another similar style diet (with some things removed/replaced) will not result in health. Fresh is always best! There is no alternative. Sorry!*

Step 5. Reintroduce foods the right way

This is also very simple. On day 24, pick **one** thing that you eliminated and eat it (for example eat eggs). Only one thing though. Everything else remains the same.

See how you feel over the next three or four days. If you have no reaction, eat the same food (in this example, eggs) again and notice how you feel. Depending on how you feel (energised after eating rather than bloated and lethargic for example) then you can decide whether or not to re-incorporate that food into your diet on a regular basis. It is about how your body 'feels' so listen to your body (your 'gut' feeling!)

After you have made the decision about the first food you reintroduced, pick another one and follow the same steps.

Throughout the diet and the reintroduction process, notice how you feel. The importance of taking the inventory at the beginning is that you may see changes that you weren't even expecting. For example, your sleep quality and your energy levels may feel better, dry red skin may have gone or improved, you may not be feeling so cold, or your tummy may stop bloating after a meal. Some people have also found that removing dairy from their diet has cured their acid reflux (Source: Dr Izabella Wentz. Thyroidpharmacist.com).

Remember that the foods in this elimination diet are the main culprits for food sensitivity, but yours could include other things, like chocolate for example (sorry!) as some foods are similar to each other in biological structure and so can cause a similar reaction in your body.

Please remember that Leaky Gut is reversible, and healing your gut, together with restoring your microbiome, can restore your health (unless most of the organ affected by the particular chronic disorder has been completely destroyed, as in Type 1 diabetes). Many chronic disorders are now being halted, and even reversed; and even people with Type 1 diabetes will benefit from finding their trigger(s) as this will prevent them from getting other autoimmune disorders and can reduce the amount of insulin they need to take.

Finally, remember that only a few weeks of change can result in a whole lifetime *without* chronic disease. You can do this!

Remember when I told you about my mum in chapter three, and I mentioned that I had given her a book about eating for your **ABO blood type**? Well, as I said there was no evidence to support it, but recent research has revealed something very interesting! Let us look again at the ABO blood type diet.

Chapter Sixteen

'ABO' Blood Type – Can it affect your gut microbiome?

I mentioned in the chapter about my mum that I had read Peter D'Adamo's books called **Eat Right 4 Your Type**, and specifically **Eat Right for Blood Type A/O/B/AB** (whatever your blood type is). He suggests that some foods are not great for us according to our blood type because of the antigens on the red blood cell surface. Although there has been no scientific research that can back this claim, there may be something in it after all, and it hasn't got anything to do with blood.

Recent research has shown that the same antigens that are on your red blood cells (that determine your ABO blood type) are also on the mucous cells in your gut. These in turn have an influence on the type and diversity of particular strains of bacteria in your gut. As we have read, diversity of gut bacteria, and also specific species of bacteria, can impact on your health and so could blood type be linked to the gut microbiome?

Other recent studies suggest that there are three 'types' of gut microbiome in human populations, and so could the ABO blood type explain this? There has not been any research in this area yet, but, nevertheless, the ABO blood type does seem to be associated with the gut microbiome, and, as different species of commensal bacteria thrive better on some food sources than others, it may be possible that food choice may indeed help people of a particular blood type, but that it has nothing to actually do with their blood!

However, recent studies showed that the **diet for blood type A was beneficial to everyone**, irrespective of their blood type! This diet includes eating only a small amount of meat and fish, no red meat, mainly vegetarian food, no wheat and no dairy and so it should be beneficial for your gut microbiome!

It also suggests not eating any of the nightshade family (potatoes, aubergines, tomatoes) as they can be inflammatory.

My tip: I mentioned this earlier, but it is worth repeating. If you are wondering what to eat if you don't eat potatoes, try parsnips. They cut up into chips and you can roast them in the oven with a little oil. They also mash well. You can do this with other root vegetables of your choice and they are all surprisingly filling!

Chapter Seventeen

Five Easy Steps – a quick guide

So we have read about the problems, the triggers and the possible solutions, and so let us summarise these into a quick guide. The main thing to remember is that chronic disorders build up over time, gradually getting worse, but if we take these five easy steps we can prevent and even reverse them.

1. **Heal the gut – diet, prebiotics, probiotics and possibly some supplements**
2. **Take measures to sustain the healthy gut – remove the food triggers.**
3. **Remove triggers other than food (where possible)**
4. **Remove stress (and how to achieve this)**
5. **Other lifestyle factors – sleep, exercise, wellbeing**

1. Heal the Gut

The first step is to heal the gut. We can do this with diet, prebiotics, probiotics, condiments and possibly some supplements. Let us start with your diet and prebiotics (which are the foods that feed your 'good' gut bacteria).

Diet and Prebiotics

Many studies show that a western diet, rich in refined starches and sugar and poor in fibre and phytonutrients from fruits and vegetables, and poor in essential fatty acids, is associated with many inflammatory disorders such as **inflammatory bowel disease, chronic asthma, rheumatoid arthritis, multiple sclerosis,**

psoriasis. Cardiovascular disease, diabetes, arthritis, and many more.

This may be because the diet may result in an excessive production of pro-inflammatory cytokines, which increase inflammation, together with a reduced production of anti-inflammatory cytokines; and this can result in **cancer**, as well as other disorders as mentioned above.

Fruit and vegetables provide the food source (soluble fibre) for your 'good' bacteria, and so they can be called prebiotics; which provide nutrients to your microbes which, in turn, contribute to your wellbeing and health. If your diet is low on these plants, you will effectively starve some of your 'good' gut bacteria, like lactobacillus, which then leaves space in your gut for other microbes to spread. Both a gut dysbiosis (lack of balance of microbes) and an overabundance of 'bad' bacteria are linked to chronic disorders (see the chapter on the gut microbiome)

Recent studies involving many plants, including onions, garlic, turmeric and ginger, show that they reduce chronic inflammation, seen in the inflammatory diseases mentioned above.

In addition, chronic inflammation is also implicated in the start of **cancer** and also the progression of **cancer**.

A diet rich in fruits and vegetables may also lower the risk of developing neurodegenerative diseases, such as **Alzheimer's disease**, because of their anti-inflammatory properties.

Rather than focus on any plant in particular here, and risk labelling it as a 'superfood', I think the message to take away from all of this is that we all need to eat a *plentiful* supply of a *variety* of different coloured fruits and vegetables (mainly vegetables).

Some of the active ingredients found in the plants may be taken in supplement form to aid health; and these were mentioned in the chapter on supplements. Supplements can be very useful, although these can never replace the fibre and other nutrients received from the whole plant.

Probiotics

We read earlier that by introducing 'good' bacteria into our gut in the form of probiotics, we will restore our microbiome to one that creates health and diminishes unhealthy cravings. A gut microbiome that is out of balance can lead to inflammation of the gut and increased permeability of the intestines; which, in turn, can lead to the development of many chronic disorders.

There are many different types available. The best ones are those that are able to survive the journey through the body without being destroyed (pharmaceutical grade), and the ones I take are by a company called Optibac because the bacteria they use were proven to work by scientific methods to date. I tried others but these worked the best for me. That being said, if you take a different brand and feel positive effects then that is fine! The thing about good bacteria is that we each have a variety of different ones, but essentially many of them have the same outcome and so don't be too worried about specific strains at first. The good bacteria that we introduce then begin to crowd out the bad microbes.

Supplements

As we know, there are things that aren't great for us in abundance, like *Candida* yeast, that we may also want to reduce in number. *Candida* are actually beneficial for us to a degree but an excess can cause the symptoms mentioned in the Elimination diet questionnaire earlier. An excess of *Candida albicans* can be treated by reducing sugar in foods and drinks and also by some supplements, like **Berberine, Saccromyces boulardi and garlic** (you can read more about this in the chapter on supplements).

2. Take Measures to Sustain the Healthy gut – Remove Food Triggers

So how do we do this? The first step is to remove the food products that are known to cause problems. These include gluten from wheat (and also barley and rye), processed sugar, dairy products (from cows milk, and also goats or sheep's milk products in some cases), eggs, soy, processed food and possibly the nightshade family (potatoes, tomatoes and aubergines). Some of you may be able to tolerate these, but if you eliminate them from your diet for at least one month, then introduce one at a time for three weeks, you will be able to feel a difference in your body if they are affecting you. The questions to ask would be those in the elimination diet.

There are many other triggers that can also cause allergic reactions, rather than sensitivity, but as your gut health improves, and consequently your immune system isn't constantly on 'high alert' you may find that some of these responses either vanish or are reduced in severity. For those that remain, there are some well documented allergens in some fruits (for example peaches), and other foods, and so eliminate them out of your diet one at a time, for a month each, and then notice if symptoms return when they are reintroduced. Obviously for very severe allergic responses just eliminate and don't re-introduce.

So, remove and/or avoid your known triggers where possible and take probiotics and any other supplements that make you feel optimal. Eat for your microbiome, by eating a variety of colours of plants. I have included some suggestions of meals to hopefully make life a little easier while you are making changes, in chapter nineteen; but how do we know if foods are good for us or not? It is possible to test, but these are often unreliable. However, there are other ways to check, and the gold standard is something called the Elimination Diet.

The Elimination diet

This is simple questionnaire which will help you know if you might need to make changes and improve your gut health.

As mentioned, if the trigger(s) remain, chronic inflammation and chronic disorder(s) persist. This can also trigger auto-immunity, where the overloaded immune system can start to make mistakes, and attack its own tissues.

A reminder that some of the triggers for **Leaky Gut** other than food might be:

Infections and gut imbalance – harmful yeasts, SIBO, and parasites.

Some medications – NSAIDS, anti-inflammatory drugs given to reduce the inflammation associated with all chronic disorders, but which can actually cause leaky gut, thereby making the condition last and make it worse over time. It may be possible to discuss alternative pain relief with your doctor.

3. Remove Non-Food Triggers (where possible)

This includes choosing shampoos, chemicals in your home, products you use in everyday life, that have as few harmful additives as possible. People ask me what I use on my hair, and I am happy to share this information, but it is not a recommendation, nor is it advice.

I use three different brands of shampoo. One is a certified organic chamomile shampoo by Urtekram, recommended to me by Roots in Sherwood, Nottingham.

The second shampoo is by Naturtint, and I also use their Nutrideep Multiplier conditioner.

The third shampoo is by PHB, and I use their Citrus and Chamomile shampoo and conditioner.

I never use air fresheners or scented candles or anything intended to disguise smells; because some of the chemicals used in them, like the fragrance limonene, become reactive once in the air, turning into the toxic chemical formaldehyde. Fresh air is the best, as it smells sweet and is also free! It isn't always easy to keep harmful products out of our lives but we are all on a journey of discovery!

4. Remove Stress and How to Achieve it

Stress, it should be remembered, is never caused by the event (what someone said or did for example), but our thoughts and responses to it. Thoughts create electrical signals in our nerves, and these trigger hormones, like cortisol, which result in emotions.

Your central nervous system communicates with your immune system via hormones, and your immune system communicates back via cytokines.

Stress response results in a release of **Cortisol**, and other stress hormones in your body, which binds to your **immune** cells and inactivates them, and also trigger **adrenaline** and so can eventually fatigue the **adrenal** system, leading to feelings of **chronic fatigue** and exhaustion, among others.

Other hormone imbalance may also cause **anxiety** (**thyroid hormones** for one).

Stress also affects the **prostaglandins** in your **digestive tract**, inhibiting them from working, which then prevents digestion of food from working properly; and this can also impact on your gut microbiome and general health.

To gain control of the effects of your alarming thoughts, a simple method is to take one or two slow breaths, while concentrating only on the breath. Push any brain chatter out of the way and keep bringing your concentration back to the slow breath. There are also some wonderful, short, meditation techniques available for free on

YouTube. Meditation doesn't have to involve sitting cross legged, holding your palms upwards while chanting! You can do a very quick meditation which just involves a few deep slow breaths as I just mentioned, or try other ways. There are so many different ones that it is possible to find one that you can relate to without feeling odd!

Another technique is to make a fist, and breathe through the small opening (adjust the size of the hole until you get just the right level of resistance for you), or breathe through a straw. This 'sucking' action fools the vagus nerve into telling your brain that you are relaxed. (It also helps people who want to stop smoking – try this instead of one of your cigarettes).

5. Other Lifestyle Factors – Sleep, Exercise and Wellbeing

Whether you call it mindfulness, conscious awareness, meditation or other forms of relaxation for your body and mind; these also contribute to a healthy body, healthy mind and healthy wellbeing. Sleep not only rests your body, it is also an opportunity for your body to provide 'housekeeping' to your brain, removing excess neurotransmitters and debris from your brain. Exercise, particularly outside, can stimulate endorphins, which make you feel good. Exercise outside also gives your body the opportunity to make vitamin D, from the sunlight hitting your skin, and make serotonin (the 'happy' hormone), from daylight hitting your hippocampus in your brain directly through your eyes. The sunlight also balances your 'body clock', making you sleepy at night and wakeful in the day.

Important

If, after three months of following all the protocols, you have not responded, you may have these additional root causes:

- Adrenal dysfunction
- Infections - for example SIBO, or parasites such as Blastocystitis (intestinal).
- Toxicity - impaired liver function

Your doctor will be able to check for these, and you may need a course of antibiotics, antifungals or antivirals before continuing on your path, but you may be able to help by undertaking a liver cleanse, to reduce any toxin burden on your liver. If you do have to take any antibiotics, Optibac have probiotics that can be taken at the same time, in order to maintain a healthy gut microbiome.

In addition, remember to eat for *your* body. If *your* body is not in optimal health and you are following a *specific* way of eating, for example paleo, vegan, and so on; then maybe try different foods and see if that helps. I am not saying that there is anything wrong with following specific ways of eating; but we are all unique and they may not work for everyone, so just be aware of that. Another thing to be aware of is that eating in a specific way may suit us at one age, say in our twenties, but that can change; as we get older or become unwell for example. The solution is to be aware and listen to *your* body.

Chapter Eighteen

Conclusion – Joining the dots

The main thing to remember is that all the different systems in your body are linked, and communicate with one another. In other words your gut microbiome, your immune system, your DNA, your digestive system, your brain and neurones, your neurotransmitters and your hormones to mention a few. These are also linked to your environment; your food and drinks, your shampoos, soaps, and antiperspirants, your exercise, your stress levels and your sleep patterns. One holistic package, where, if one system has a problem it impacts on all the rest; so we need to address all of them, and not just focus on the one thing that seems to be the problem.

There is a preponderance of scientific evidence to show that eating a diet consisting mainly of plants, preferably organic, with either little or no animal protein, again preferably organic or wild, is beneficial to the health of our gut bacteria, and so consequently beneficial to our own health; leading to a healthy body, healthy mind, healthy weight and healthy wellbeing. Having a healthy gut, with mainly good bacteria, leads to a healthy gut lining (free of leaky gut) and, also importantly, a healthy immune system, which in turn protects us from invading viruses and bacteria, and also reduces allergic responses. The diversity and quantity of bacterial strains are also essential for life, and we read, in the chapter on the gut microbiome, how many different functions the gut bacteria have. In addition, other triggers in our environment that we *can* control, particularly those in our own home, can be reduced, as we have control over what we spray on our furniture or put on our body; and this in turn reduces our 'toxic burden'.

We can never be in control of everything around us, and we shouldn't even worry about that as the stress of doing so would undo all the good that we have done by eating healthily and making sure our gut microbiome is healthy! Some viruses and toxins in the air, or air pollution, may also be potential triggers, but we can't remove all things which may do us harm, and there is no need to panic about this. If we take care of our gut, maintain a healthy microbiome, keeping it in balance, this will then create and maintain a healthy gut immune system, which will be much better able to fight and destroy potentially harmful things which we come into contact with. However, if all of the protocols you are taking are not removing these infections then your doctor will be able to recommend medications needed; for example antivirals or antifungals; or even antibiotics if necessary. Functional medicine doctors are saying that many of their patients find that once they get their gut microbiome into 'balance', other problems simply go away. This, of course is anecdotal, but there will not be any study undertaken which wants to prove that you can take your health into your own hands, not take expensive (profitable) drugs, and not eat (profitable) 'food' that comes with a list of additives and preservatives in the ingredients. However, some medications are both necessary and optimal and so the main thing to remember is that we work together with our doctors. This book is to help us to follow paths to heal ourselves, but it is also necessary to work with your doctor, to keep track of antibodies and other autoimmune and chronic disorder markers for example. So it is up to each of us, as individuals, to tune into our bodies, and feed it what it needs (healthy whole foods) rather than what the brain is directed to 'want' from 'bad' bugs in our gut, or from advertisements, or from 'reward' impulses from the brain, triggered by processed foods, artificial substances and processed drinks. We also need to take some exercise, get enough sleep, eat slowly and mindfully, manage stress and make time for fun with people we like and love. Importantly, also learn to love ourselves, leaving situations and people if they aren't good for us.

You are unique. You can do this!

Things that we have considered throughout this book, and dots that we have joined, include:

- Your genes and how big a part they play in chronic disorders
- How epigenetic markers on our DNA can be inherited; and reversed
- Your environment and how big a part it plays in chronic disorders
- Your gut microbiome
- How your gut microbiome can be out of balance
- The effect of antibiotics on your gut microbiome
- Why gut microbes are necessary for life
- Balancing your gut microbiome, and restoring it to health
- Links between your gut microbiome and your immune system
- How your immune system creates chronic disorders
- Your digestive system
- Diet - food triggers for chronic disorders and effects on the gut
- Information about processed food and how quickly it has evolved
- The difference between sea salt (natural, has added minerals) and table salt (man-made sodium chloride)
- The difference between sugar found in fruit and vegetables, and table sugar (extracted from plants, and rapidly absorbed by your body).
- Why the rapid absorption of some processed foods can cause chronic disorders.

- How food can affect our DNA – epigenetics
- How food can influence your grandchildren - epigenetics
- Prebiotics – food for your gut microbes; which are essential for your health and wellbeing (producing vitamins and neurotransmitters among others)
- Probiotics – to restore and heal the gut and also preventing and reversing chronic disorders.
- Leaky gut repair preventing chronic disorders
- Gut inflammation – links to hormones like ghrelin and leptin, the gut and the immune system.
- Links between adipose tissue (fat cells), gut inflammation and obesity
- Autoimmunity
- Autoimmunity as a continuum
- Infections
- Non-food triggers and how you can manage your own environment
- Feeding your restored and healthy microbiome to keep it healthy; and how that reverses and prevents chronic disorders
- Links between your gut and your brain; and how you can prevent and reverse disorders thought to be confined to the brain
- Gut microbes can influence your thoughts and food preferences
- Gut microbes can alter your taste sensors so that you like what they want you to eat
- You are in ultimate control, not your gut microbes, which are replaced every twenty four hours or so.
- Links between food triggers, Leaky Gut and Leaky Brain

- Links between food triggers and 'brain' disorders like mood, anxiety, depression, autism, ADHD and Alzheimer's disease.
- Why we have two 'brains' and how they interact with each other
- Links between stress, your microbiome and your immune system; and how you can reduce stress
- Why stress causes digestion problems
- How some probiotics can reduce the chances of getting a cold
- Links between **all** chronic disorders and how to prevent and, in many cases, reverse them.
- Why the link between all chronic disorders means that having one chronic disorder means you are much more likely to get another
- Why finding your trigger(s) can prevent you from getting other chronic disorders, and heal and possibly reverse the one(s) you already have.
- Spices and condiments can aid healing
- How hormones are linked to what you eat, digest and absorb
- How hormones are affected by diet and lifestyle; and how they impact on chronic disorders
- That thoughts create electrical signals in our nerves, which trigger hormones; which in turn create emotions
- How science may explain the 'ego'
- How curiosity calms our 'default mode network' (mind chatter)
- Why 'mind chatter' is a survival mode
- How other factors, including meditation and mindfulness reduce stress levels and improve sleep

• Why sleep is important for physical and mental health, and how daylight increases your feel good hormones (serotonin), sets your body clock (produces melatonin), helps you to make vitamin D (needed for bones and your immune system) and improves your wellbeing

• Exercise improves physical and mental health, and it doesn't have to be at a gym.

Take home summary

I wrote myself a summary to help me join the dots, and so I share this with you here:

1. Always get a diagnosis from your doctor rather than self-diagnose.

2. Get any medications needed to an optimal level that is working for you.

3. Antibiotics and some medications; a typical western diet high in carbohydrates and low in vegetables, missing meals, and stress, lead to:

4. A dysbiosis in the gut microbiome, blood sugar spikes, reduced vitamins and minerals, and increased levels of cortisol which leads to:

5. Impaired digestion and food movement through the intestines, leaky gut, food intolerances, nutrient-deficiency in the body, immune overload, an impact on the liver and adrenal glands and inflammation.

6. As this progresses it can lead to an increase in many symptoms, and possibly raised antibodies; resulting finally in a chronic disorder and possibly an autoimmune disorder.

7. Work together with your doctor to keep tabs on diagnostic markers of a disorder. You may need to take antivirals, antifungals or other medication.

Three further points to note:

8. If, after eating a nutrient rich whole food diet, and following protocols suggested for three months, symptoms or diagnostic markers (from samples, for example blood samples, taken by your doctor) still remain, then it may be worth trying a liver cleanse. This is because the elimination of toxins starts in the gut, but then, if the gut is inflamed or overloaded, the toxins pass to the liver, which may then become overloaded and congested.

9. Your stress levels impact your adrenal glands which also affect your cortisol levels. Eventually cortisol levels drop. However, because cortisol is anti-inflammatory this can be unhelpful. Adrenal hormones also drop which can lead to feelings of exhaustion. For these reasons, stress management is needed for physical, as well as mental, wellbeing.

10. If you follow a particular 'diet' or lifestyle and you are still having symptoms, then listen to your body, rather than follow a suggested way of living. We are all unique.

The desire to control our environment has led to an illusion of 'separateness'; 'fighting' things that appear to be 'bad' or 'wrong'. The discovery of the microbiome returns us to a more holistic view, of co-operation, working together for optimal health and wellbeing. We can extend this out to nature, our food, other people, other living things and our environment; removing boundaries.

Rather than fighting our body, or nature; if we use the information in this book as a guide, we can work with them; thinking of symptoms as a helpful clue as to how we have deviated from health, rather than something to fear or fight against.

Making changes can lead to:

- A strengthened immune system
- Reduced inflammation

- Controlling the expression of your genes
- Improving your metabolism
- Controlling the amount of calories you absorb
- Improving your mood and anxiety levels
- Increasing your wellbeing

All leading to:

- A healthy body, healthy weight, and healthy mind!

TAKE HOME MESSAGE

Your plan

The purpose of this book is to achieve a healthy body, healthy weight and healthy mind (and, I will also include, a healthy wellbeing!) in five easy steps, so let us remind ourselves of the five step plan.

Five-step plan

1.   Re-inoculate your gut microbiome (as some essential bacteria are killed off with antibiotics, other medication that you may have taken, increased stress and dietary changes).

2.   Feed the healthy microbiome, taking supplements where needed.

3.   Remove food triggers to restore your gut to health.

4.   Avoid non-food triggers where possible.

5.   Take steps to get enough sleep and exercise, and manage stress.

So how do we achieve those? Let us have a quick reminder:

Probiotics – taken to restore an imbalance in your gut microbiome. This impacts on physical and mental health and also on wellbeing, as gut bacteria make things like serotonin, the 'happy' hormone, and many vitamins essential for health (among other things). A balanced microbiome also leads to a balanced weight.

Prebiotics – to feed your gut microbiome, which in turn keeps us healthy. Both prebiotic food and probiotics enhance the barrier function in the intestines, blood capillaries and elsewhere; leading to reduced inflammation and a strengthened immune system. This also keeps hormones in balance, and this is essential for physical and mental health and wellbeing. It will also balance your weight.

Eat organic food where possible – but don't stress if you can't. Eat mainly vegetables, as they feed your gut microbiome, and, if you eat them, eat only small amounts of organic meat or wild fish (avoiding those with mercury). Avoid pesticides and herbicides where possible, as 'foreign' chemicals can be a trigger that contributes towards health problems. We are lucky in the EU, as we have fantastic regulations that keep our food relatively safe to eat. This does not apply everywhere.

Supplements if needed – to **restore** balance of minerals, vitamins and enhance healing.

Medication if needed – to aid healing.

No processed foods or drinks including processed sugar and salt because they contribute to health problems. (Alternative: fruit and sea salt)

Remove food triggers – Take an **elimination diet** (dairy, wheat gluten, egg, processed foods and soy are common triggers) to find your food triggers. We are all unique so this is the gold standard. If yours is not one of the common triggers, keep eliminating one of your regular foods until you find it. Removing triggers removes an immune response with associated inflammation, gut dysbiosis and hormone imbalances,

Eating – times of day (not late evening, as your body's cortisol levels are at their highest in the morning, and so eating later is more likely to cause weight gain); and **speed of eating** (slowly and mindfully) improves digestion and achieves possible weight loss or weight gain if needed. Weight loss can also be achieved simply by removing processed foods like sugar and eating to feed your gut microbiome. Different foods also affects our mood and wellbeing either positively or negatively (nutritious food or junk food).

Avoid non-food triggers – for example air fresheners, cleaning chemicals (alternative, use baking soda in a little water), air pollution and scented candles (fragrance can become toxic in the air). The reason we want to avoid as many triggers of poor health as possible is to give our body a better chance of healing and repairing itself. Remember that long term health problems do not start overnight; but are on a continuum. If we overload our body with many different triggers, it will struggle to keep us healthy. Saying that, your body has a miraculous ability to heal itself, but it can only cope with so much before it buckles under.

Sleep – set your body clock (get 30 minutes of daylight a day to set yours. It can be taken in chunks of five or ten minutes), and limit use of TV/mobile phone/tablet late at night (blue light induces wakefulness). Sleep allows 'housekeeping' in your brain to remove excess neurotransmitters and other waste products. This is helpful in the prevention of disorders of the brain like Alzheimer's disease. Aim to be asleep by 11pm, as your hormones and digestive system work in cinque with daylight hours.

Exercise - 30 minute walk most days if possible, but at least three times a week – exercise releases 'feel-good' endorphins, your skin will make vitamin D from the sunlight (which is needed for your immune system and bones) and you can be aware of your senses, aware of the present moment (which reduces anxiety and calms 'mind-chatter'). It also calms an overworked adrenal system, which, when pushed, results in constant tiredness but an inability to sleep.

Stress – relaxation, exercise, walking (outside – sunlight causes your skin to make vitamin D, and you also set your body clock; producing melatonin to improve sleep) and meditation (being mindful, being aware of the present moment and not being distracted by thoughts that take you elsewhere). Stress impacts on your adrenal system (which can leave you feeling fatigued), immune system (reducing your ability to fight disease), digestion (reducing your ability to absorb essential nutrients) and many hormones; and so getting back into balance can help most health problems.

Key elements of chronic and autoimmune disorders - The key elements involved in the process of **inflammation, chronic disorders, allergies, asthma, autoimmunity,** and **cancer**, are now known to include:

1. Genetic predisposition (which plays a minor role),
2. Exposure to environmental triggers and epigenetics (which play a major role and are reversible and preventable), and
3. Leaky Gut, caused by activation of the zonulin pathway due to:

    Food triggers and/or

    Changes in the gut microbiome

The key systems mentioned throughout this book all contribute towards long term health.

The good news is that the constant interplay between your gut microbiome, your genes and the environment, means that although a chronic disease process may start, it can be modified or even reversed. For the *first* time, we have innovative management solutions for what were considered to be incurable debilitating diseases.

Breaking news!!

The breaking news is that some new and exciting research involving eight hundred people published in November 2015, investigating high blood glucose levels, proved a link between chronic disorders and our microbiome.

In this research they showed how different gut bacteria can mean the difference between health and chronic disorder, being lean or obese, having high cholesterol or not and so on.

The study, which is ongoing, looks at people in their normal environments, eating the food they normally eat, eating in their normal way, looking at the times of day that they eat, their lifestyle and their environment; and this one piece of research links with, and supports what I have written about in this book.

Even more exciting is that the study found that certain changes can improve the markers of chronic disorders in only a few days!!

Breaking news

On 13 April 2016, the European Parliament voted to ban most uses of glyphosate (active ingredient of the weed killer Roundup ™); including pre-harvest application on crops, and using in or around public parks and playgrounds. This overturned the decision by the European Commission to extend the use of glyphosate for fifteen years without restrictions; but is not binding on Member States at this time. The EU governments will discuss this partial ban further, possibly in May 2016. The banning of glyphosate, until proven safe, receives support from two thirds of European citizens.

Remember: Your body has a miraculous ability to heal itself.

There will always be viruses and genetic mutations which beat us, but if we can take as many harmful things out of our personal environment as possible, and eat and use as many healthy things as possible, with as healthy a lifestyle as possible, then the future will certainly be lots brighter!

Your future from here

You may feel a resistance to some of the things in this book at first, as our (default mode network) minds can become very resistant to change; but the choice is yours, and the tools to do it are in this book and other resources. You are in control of you, and you can choose your path through life. It can be healthy and joyful, with normal ups and down of life (although even those ups and downs can be viewed differently if we don't follow every thought). I know you will make the right choice for you, and whatever that may be I wish you love and hugs, and all the best wishes in the world to achieve your goals.

The next chapter includes some food ideas to start you on your journey, but I will leave you with this:

Your body's miraculous ability to heal is greater than anyone has ever permitted you to believe. I think that is possibly the best take home message we could ever have. ☺

Susie xo

Chapter Nineteen

Some new ways of eating – meal ideas

The thing about meals, for me, is to make it as easy as possible! I make double or triple amounts of things and put them in the freezer, ready for lazy or busy days.

Breakfasts

Fresh seaweed with rice noodles, pak choi, vegetable stock and organic miso paste (or organic tamari, which is a wheat free soy sauce)

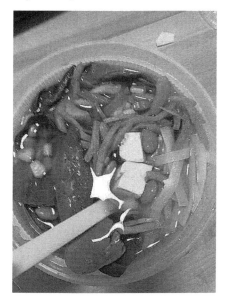

I buy my seaweed from Bute in Scotland, and it is delicious!! My research taught me that nori (purple larva), including the dried nori (which changes it from purple to green with no effect) is an excellent source of Vitamin B12 (only normally found in animal products) and also iodine and many other minerals and vitamins that we need.

The meal smells like the sea and always makes me feel happy!

Essentially, in a wok, or deep frying pan, add a little oil (I use sesame or olive oil), then

Fry some spring onions,

Add the chopped pak choi, then the

Beansprouts,

Carrots

Celery

Organic beans of choice (for example cannellini beans)

Tofu (optional)

Add the stock and miso paste (or tamari), rice noodles, and finally

The seaweed.

Heat though for a few minutes and then serve!! (Strangely, my body doesn't react badly to (organic) soy sauce but it does to (organic) tofu. I don't know why but like finding all other food triggers, it is trial and error, combined with an elimination diet!)

Alternatives: You could use kale or other leafy vegetables instead of, or as well as, the pak choi. If you eat meat you could use a chicken stock. You can add organic tofu if you can eat soy products.

I eat this for breakfast as well as for lunch or dinner! I realised that it is only tradition that stops us from eating certain foods at certain times. Many countries eat vegetables for breakfast, and they are a yummy start to the day!

Smoothie

Now I don't always have these for breakfast because I prefer to eat whole foods rather than blend lots together, but many people adore them so I am including them here as a breakfast idea (for those reluctant to try my seaweed breakfast!). If you have a blender use soft leafy green vegetables and salad, like kale and spinach, and add things of your choice. Beetroot is nice, and you can sweeten it with some fruit. Juices, rather than smoothies, remove all of the soluble fibre that your microbiome needs, and also gives you a rapid supply of fruit sugar, and so I am not a fan of juices. You can buy blenders now that can blend almost anything! If you do buy one, like a Vitamix for example, make sure that you hear it working before you buy it, as they can be terribly noisy! Also, there are different shaped ones (wide based, narrow based), depending on what you want to use them for.

Almond milk

You can also use the blender to make your own 'milk', like almond milk for example. You blend the almonds with water then strain it through a cloth. Again, I am not a huge fan of discarding the remaining nut pulp and so would recommend using this somewhere if possible. I am not a fan of any 'milk' alternative and so don't use it, but if you want to drink almond milk with your cereal, this is a great way to do it.

Organic blueberries with organic figs and organic prunes

One of my favourite breakfasts is organic blueberries with organic figs and organic prunes (partly dried. You can buy them from Sainsbury's and health stores); followed by a slice of gluten free bread, with a little sunflower spread (and either organic hummus or something sweet of your choice). You could add a sliced or mashed banana to the bread.

Porridge

If you like porridge there are many 'milks' available as an alternative to dairy, or you can mix the organic oats with a choice of organic cranberries, organic raisins, organic figs and organic prunes. Delicious!

Muesli

I also make my own easy peasy organic gluten free muesli, and keep it in a tub. Essentially it is a combination of:

Oats,

Chopped Brazil nuts

Walnuts,

Cranberries,

Raisins,

Sliced almonds,

Sesame seeds and

Poppy seeds.

Shake it all up and it doesn't need any 'milk'. It is delicious and moist just on its own.

Alternatives

You can experiment with the muesli by using different seeds and nuts and fruit, making different ones each time. You can add fruit to your porridge. There are also 'meat alternatives' available, like vegan bacon and vegan sausages. I am not a huge fan of processed food so do not eat these but they are an alternative to animal bacon and sausages if that is what you prefer. You can also buy gluten free sausages (Sainsbury's sell them in their freezer section) and many other delicious alternatives.

Easy peasy gluten free bread

I use the recipe on the back of Doves Farm organic gluten free bread flour, and it is so easy it is unbelievable! I changed it slightly as I use honey or agave nectar instead of sugar, and I don't use the egg alternative. The flour can be bought in many health food stores and in Sainsburys supermarket.

Even easier is the organic, yeast free, gluten free, seeded bread mix by Amisa; that you simply mix with water and bake in the oven for 60 minutes!

If you eat eggs, you could have a boiled (organic free range) egg with gluten free toast and sunflower spread (the brand 'Pure' say that they do not use emulsifiers). You could also make scrambled egg, with the toast, and you can add spinach on the side if you fancy it!

If you eat bread that is not gluten free, try to eat organic bread, as this wheat has not been sprayed with glyphosate. You may find, if you take the elimination test, that you can tolerate organic bread but not non-organic bread.

Lunches and Dinners

Bubble and Squeak – in bulk!

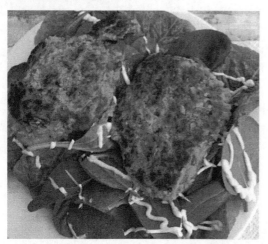

One of my favourites is a 'bubble and squeak', where I cook a variety of green vegetables (ones you like), plus carrots, suede, potatoes and sweet potatoes and onion.

Simply cook all of the green vegetables in one pan, all of the others (except the onion) in a second pan, and fry the chopped onions in a frying pan.

Mash the potato mixture, season with salt, pepper and herbs of your choice. Roughly cut up the green vegetables and add to the potato mixture. Add the fried onions.

Form into potato cakes (the shape of scones), and place on a chopping board to cool.

Place two at a time in a food bag and put into the freezer.

When you want to eat them, defrost and then place on a baking tray at 175 degrees (fan oven) for around twenty minutes, until hot with a crispy brown surface.

Eat either alone, or with other steamed vegetables, or with salad, or meat if you eat it. It is also nice with a sauerkraut (made with salt not vinegar). It is a fantastic prebiotic too!

Alternatives:

Make the potato cakes with different vegetables, like beetroot, mushrooms, spinach or whatever you fancy really. Experiment! You can use less potato and add quinoa or rice. Also you can make it into a burger, and eat with a gluten free bread roll and salad.

Pan fried tofu with sweet potato mash, green beans, gluten free gravy and mixed seeds of your choice

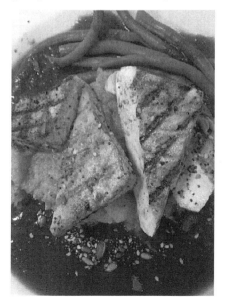

Vegetable and bean casserole (makes about six bowls)

One of my favourites!

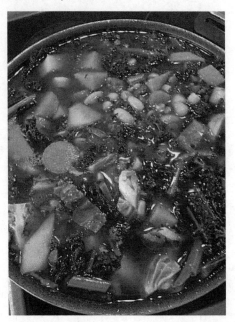

You can make this with any vegetables that you have in your store cupboard; particularly if they need using up. Try a mixture of carrots, parsnips, squash, onions, garlic, green vegetables and beans. My favourite so far is the following mixture. They are all organic and most of them are from Abel and Cole.

Parsnips (about six)

Carrots (about four)

Brussel sprouts (about twelve)

Onions (about three)

Garlic (two cloves)

Kale (about three big handfuls)

Tin of sweetcorn

Carton of organic cannellini beans

Carton of organic chopped tomatoes

Carton of organic black beans

Two tablespoons of Sainsburys reduced salt yeast extract

Fresh thyme (leaves only, a couple of sprigs)

Organic herbs de provence (or herb mixture of your choice).

Tablespoon of olive oil

Method:

Chop all vegetables and place in a large heated pan with the olive oil. I generally start with the onion and fry that off a bit and then add the others, as I've chopped them, just throwing it all in together!

Fill with filtered water and add the yeast extract and herbs.

Bring to the boil and then place in a low oven (it should be simmering slowly) for a few hours.

Take out of the pan and place into large Pyrex glass bowls to cool. Place in fridge (or put some in the freezer for a lazy meal instead of a takeaway).

Aubergine and Patatas Bravas (feeds two)

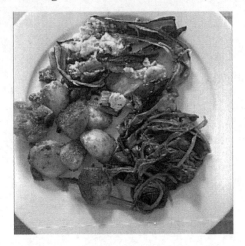

Potatoes (as many as two people want to eat)

Aubergine

Spinach

Chilli powder (a teaspoon)

Smoked paprika (a teaspoon)

Olive oil

Feta cheese (optional)

Method:

Boil the potatoes and cool slightly. Add the chilli powder and paprika and cat the potatoes.

Slice the aubergine long ways and brush with olive oil. Place in a frying pan with a little oil and fry until golden brown.

At the same time, put a tablespoon of olive oil in a wok, heat until very hot and add the potatoes coated in chilli and paprika. Cook on high heat until crispy on the surface and heated all the way through.

Steam the spinach until slightly wilted. Serve with the aubergine and potatoes (and feta cheese if using)!

Broccoli and Butternut Squash with Rocket and Roast Pumpkin Seeds

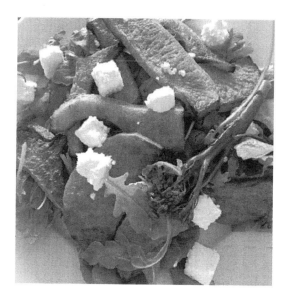

Peel and slice the butternut squash and coat in a little olive oil. Place on a baking tray and roast in the oven until slightly brown). Place pumpkin seeds on a baking tray and place in the oven for one or two minutes (they burn very quickly so take care).

Steam the broccoli and add to the butternut squash. Serve with rocket and a drizzle of olive oil. Sprinkle with roast pumpkin seeds. For people who eat cheese, you could add feta cheese crumbled over this.

Jacket potato / Chunky organic healthy chips

I love to eat this and it is a real standby meal for me. I use sunflower spread by Pure and then either organic hummus, or organic baked beans, with rocket and maybe beetroot and organic butterbeans. Or you can make your own organic chunky chips, by coating the potato chips in a little olive oil, placing them on a baking tray and place in a preheated oven, at 170 degrees (fan oven) for thirty minutes (or until golden brown).

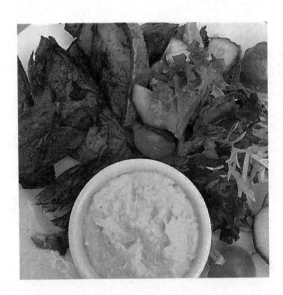

Veggie Burger

You can boil some sweet potato and mash it, and then add whatever you fancy. I've tried mushrooms, spinach, beetroot, onions, cannellini beans, broccoli and cauliflower in various combinations and they are all delicious! After you have made it, let it cool and then place on a baking tray in the oven until it is crispy and slightly brown. Yum! Eat on their own or with salad.

Other ideas:

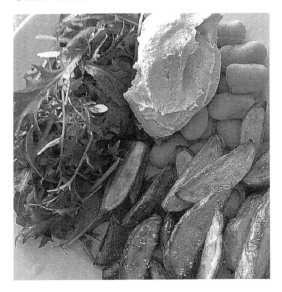

Gluten Free Penne Pasta

You can fry onions, garlic, green beans, broccoli, tomatoes, cannellini beans and red peppers in a wok and then add the mixture to the cooked penne. Quick, easy and delicious!

Roast chunks of root vegetables with quinoa

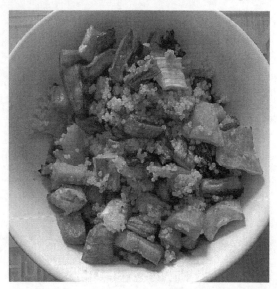

Ingredients

Carrots, suede, and any vegetables of your choice. I included asparagus in this one.

Pine nuts

Olive oil

Method

Cut up the vegetables into large chunks, place in a bowl and drizzle with oil. Place on a baking tray, in a preheated oven, 170 degrees (fan oven), for about thirty minutes (until golden brown).

About ten minutes from the end of cooking time, add two parts of boiling water to one part quinoa in a pan. Cover, and simmer until the water has been absorbed by the quinoa (about five minutes).

Mix together and serve. (This could be eaten hot or cold, with rocket and pine nuts).

Alternative

Pan-fry sliced courgettes and onions, and add these to the quinoa instead of the roasted root vegetables. Sprinkle with pine nuts and olive oil and serve with rocket.

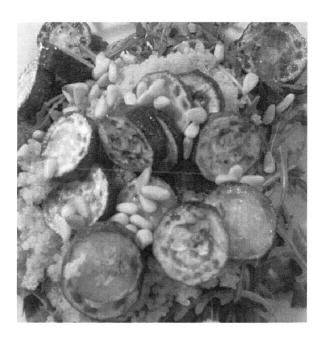

Light lunch idea – Avocado, Red Grapefruit and pomegranate

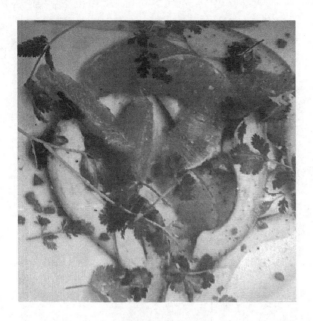

Ingredients and Method

Half an organic avocado, sliced

Half a red grapefruit in segments

Pomegranate seeds sprinkled over

Garnish with flat leaf parsley and olive oil

Puddings

I don't usually have a pudding as I don't really have a sweet tooth, but sometimes will have a frozen coconut milk yoghurt (chocolate or plain) by coconut collaborative. They are just like ice cream and are delicious!! I add raisins and pine nuts occasionally for a change.

Coconut Collaborative also make yoghurt made with coconut milk and they are delicious too. Don't be put off by the natural ones, as they are sweet and delicious (and not at all sour like the milk ones).

All of Coconut Collaborative products also have probiotics in them and prebiotic inulin so they are actually a healthy pudding! Win win! You could have fruit of course, but there are lots of recipes out there, in vegan food magazines or other healthy magazines or online, to tempt your taste buds!

Drinks

The secret to drinking alcohol is to have a very small glass of it, with food. Anything more is a poison. Sorry!

Other than that, it is best to drink only water with your meal, as it is refreshing, it quenches your thirst, it hydrates you and it has zero calories.

Sugary drinks just add calories, and will make you feel hungry afterwards as they spike your insulin levels, which then makes your blood sugar temporarily low and sends hunger signals to your brain. Before you dismiss this, and say that you enjoy your fizzy drink, remember that only 100 extra calories a day can add 14 pounds of weight a year!

Coffee and tea are fine in moderation, but too much caffeine can exhaust your adrenal glands. Green tea is supposed to be better for us than black tea.

Finally

Life is a journey, so try different foods and experiment with new tastes. Feel great knowing that each *whole* food that you eat adds to your health and happiness. Eating the right foods will leave you feeling energised, well and joyful. You can do this! I know that you will make the right choices for you. Remember to be patient with yourself and be kind to yourself. If you slip back to old habits, just start again with the very next meal.

This is your journey towards a healthy body, healthy weight, healthy mind and healthy wellbeing; and I wish you love and hugs xo

Appendix 1

My Personal Protocol

My foods

People ask me what I eat, and so this section is really to share just that, but I don't intend any of them as a recommendation, but just ideas that you may or may not wish to try for yourselves.

Essentially I eat all of the things in chapter nineteen, with more besides, eating whole foods in the main. A simple rule is, if you can pick it, eat it, if it is made in a factory, don't eat it! Saying that there are a few exceptions to my rule, like the organic Be'ond bars, Vego chocolate, and I love 'Violife' 'cheddar' slices made from coconut oil. I use these rarely though, and my diet is normally fresh produce.

I have also changed my thoughts on breakfast. We have all become so used to eating certain food types at breakfast, but now I eat vegetables, and salads. A large casserole pot of organic vegetables and beans, together with Sainsbury's reduced salt yeast extract (like Marmite but less salt) is both easy and delicious! (See the chapter on recipes for an idea of which vegetables to use together). Fresh seaweed, with beansprouts and onion with a little organic tamari (soy sauce) is a particularly yummy breakfast as it is so light and fresh! People in other cultures eat this way, so it is just a matter of changing old habits. Dried Nori, soaked for a few seconds in water, is a great alternative to fresh seaweed.

After eating whole foods, and avoiding processed foods (even vegan and vegetarian processed foods) in the main, I feel healthy and energised, because of the combination of a change in my diet and lifestyle, together with ten minutes of being aware each day (a good question to ask yourself is 'Where am I right now, what can I see, smell, hear?' and just be aware of your present moment). Both my body and my mind feel in tune with one another and I feel mentally and physically relaxed and joyful (not that I am without challenges, but I have an inner 'joy', which is different to fleeting 'happiness').

My 'meditation' or 'awareness' or 'mindfulness' has also (almost) got rid of stress created by thought, as I no longer follow thoughts other than those which are practical and useful or essential. Maybe because of this, and also because I take probiotics which may have altered my urges for particular drinks and foods, I no longer feel a strong desire for alcohol; although I do have an occasional glass of champagne, or cherry kirsch, or Cointreau. One of my favourite cocktails for summer is a mojito as it is so refreshing, and my favourite cocktail of all time is a raspberry 75, introduced to me by the wonderful Fairmont MacDonald hotel in Alberta, Canada. It is a combination of half a shot of Absolut vodka, with freshly pureed raspberry, topped up with (Moet et Chandon) champagne. Yum!

My sweet desire is solved by fine dark chocolates and there are some delicious ones, made in England too! My favourites are Seed & Bean, stocked by The Chocolate Shop in Southwell Nottinghamshire which has some of the best chocolate ever (including non-soy vegan chocolate)!! Other choices include Vego, one of the most delicious nut vegan chocolates ever, which I buy from Roots, a wonderful shop in Sherwood Nottingham, who stock the most amazing range of healthy, vegan, organic foods and supplements.

My non-foods

I use cruelty free products wherever possible, and also ones with as few chemicals in as possible. I also support small businesses as they are the lifeline of a country. It is good to bear in mind that just because something is 'natural' it doesn't make it safe or harmless.

Aloe makes my skin itchy for example. It is a case of trial and error, to see which products suit you best, but I use the following:

Shampoo Brands - Naturetint; PHB (Citrus and Chamomile) and Urtekram (Camomile).

Conditioner Brands – Naturetint (Nutrideep Multiplier) and PHB (Citrus and Chamomile)

My probiotics

I mentioned earlier, in the chapter on probiotics, that I use those from a company called Optibac, as their probiotics are pharmaceutical grade, and are backed by scientific research. I stay using them because the strains that they use are effective for me, and I no longer get asthma or react to dust. If I do get a cold it is minor and I heal very quickly.

As I mentioned, I use their 'Extra Strength Every Day' probiotics, as they stop me getting asthma and allergies, and seem to boost my immune system, but we are all unique and so other strains may be useful for you.

They do make one which is specific for people taking antibiotics as they are not killed by the antibiotic and so can be taken at the same time, which may be useful.

My supplements

I use liquorice root and glutamine to heal my gut, and occasionally use *saccromyces boulardii*, a yeast which removes some of the excess *Candida* from your gut, and CandidaStat (a combination of garlic, berberine and more) as these are thought to help balance the amount of Candida albicans in our gut. The latter two stop me getting urges for sugar and also stop the symptoms of *Candida* overload and so I'm presuming that they work, but can't offer any scientific proof, as supplements are rarely tested in trials. They are recommended by many functional medicine doctors and practitioners however.

My exercise routine

I used to do aerobics, but now I prefer to do a four mile hilly walk (just around my neighbourhood), three or four times a week, and do weight exercises at home, recommended in the 'Biggest Loser' book (they have professional trainers). For anyone who struggles with exercise because of bad backs, joints or pelvic floor weakness, there are exercises tips available to help. Walking outside is my 'meditation' too.

My weight

My weight, which was never an issue until I reached my late forties, has been normalised by the changes in my diet, and the weights I use for resistance exercises keep my body strong and toned.

Prior to making the changes in my diet and lifestyle (removing triggers) it didn't matter what exercise I did, and how careful I was with my food, I could not lose weight very easily.

I have never been an overweight person, but put weight on when I was in my late forties. Everyone blames the menopause for this, and a change in hormones can certainly have an effect on weight, but I also knew women who had not gained weight and so I knew that it couldn't be just that.

I know that we lose muscle mass after about the age of forty, and as muscle is very good at burning calories this could have been one reason for my weight gain, but even exercise didn't help so I had my doubts about that.

I suspect that my thyroid gland may not have been working optimally (despite TSH tests which said that it was fine), and that by removing gluten and dairy this then returned to health, although that is just my personal opinion.

The changes in my diet and lifestyle (I followed my own advice!) was made in conjunction with taking the probiotic I mentioned above, and this brought my gut microbiome back into balance. As we have said throughout the book, the measures I took gave my whole body the ability to regain balance and start to heal itself. I now feel healthy and fit and am back to a dress size 10!

My meditation and attitude to life

There have been many influences on my life (as well as my wonderful family and friends) which have changed my view of life. These include my yoga teacher, at the age of fifteen, who said "Don't say unpleasant things about another person". She went on to say "I know what you're thinking, you're thinking, but I have to say it because I'm thinking it, and it will drive me crazy to keep it to myself. So the answer is, don't think the thoughts". Very profound, and she started me on the long journey of realising that thoughts can be ignored.

Although I did put my yoga teacher's advice into practice at the time, I truly understood and felt the change in my body and mind, as a result of not following every thought, years later, after listening to Eckhart Tolle and Oprah Winfrey's worldwide webcasts, where they discussed each chapter of 'A new Earth', and answered questions live from people around the world. It was when he said that he reached a low point and thought "I can't live with myself" that he stopped, and thought "that sounds like there are two of me!" Essentially he realised that there was him, and then there were his thoughts (constant mind chatter, not the practical thoughts we need for everyday life) which are negative and often fearful; always either about the past or the future. He also realised that these thoughts always take you away from the present moment, the 'now' (which is what he means by 'The Power of Now', another book of his); and that if we follow mind chatter then we are never actually present, here and now, as our thoughts are taking us either to the past or the future!

I won't say too much more about this, but one thing I found really useful was if a thought keeps going round and round in your head (going over a problem of some sort) and you can't stop it; Eckhart Tolle suggests asking yourself the question "do I have that problem right now?" and then observe, without labelling anything with a thought, what there is right now. For example, if you are sitting in your car what can you see? Maybe you can see the trees, the sun is shining and people are walking by, doing their shopping. That is what is happening right now. Anything else is just a thought. Right now is 'what is'. Right now I don't have a problem (that I am thinking of). Right now, I'm just sitting in my car!

He explains that stress occurs when what you want is different to what is. For example, if you are sitting in your car but want to be at home. Thoughts which tell you that you don't want to be in your car will make you unhappy or cross or stressed. What they can never do, however, is change the situation (what is). You are in your car, no matter what thoughts your mind creates! His solution is to accept the present moment and then do one of three things.

- **The first** is always to accept the reality of what is, as it is what it is. In our example, the reality is that you are sitting in your car.
- **The second** is to see if you can change your situation (can you leave your car for example). If you can make the change that you want, then do it.
- **The third**, if you cannot change your situation, is to accept that you can't make the change right now (although you can make plans for a change) and just be present (being

aware of what is happening right now). In this example, accept that you are in your car until you get home!

That way, there is no additional layer of stress or unhappiness. It takes some practice, and it may only last for a minute at first, but it gets easier and easier to do. If a negative/complaining/fearful thought comes into my head now, I don't react to it as I once would have done. Those thoughts have lost their power in other words, and life is joyful. Still with challenges, but joyful, as the extra layer of stress (produced by thoughts) has gone.

Mindfulness

Very recently, I found another book that is very useful in putting the daily practice of awareness, or mindfulness, into practice, and that is one called 'Practical Mindfulness by Ken A. Verni Psy.D. He gives useful tips and guidance that you can use in your everyday life.

Finally, I recently bought an amazing mindfulness album called Self-Care for Busy People. You can buy it online and download it to your laptop, tablet or phone. There are ten tracks, and they take from four to twelve minutes, for all times of the day. Kris has an amazingly soothing voice, and she even knows that our mind is being distracted; wondering when the track will finish! It helps you reduce stress and increase inner calm and joy. See http://kriscarr.com for details of how to buy it.

Science supports mindfulness

As a scientist, to know that this pattern of thinking or feeling is backed up by physical activity in different parts of our brain, helps me put the spiritual 'abstract' feelings into a more grounded 'logical' thought process, which I find helpful; not because I have difficulty grasping the abstract, but because I find 'survival' mode a more pleasant concept to recognise in others than a rather self-centred 'egoic' mode.

The science behind it lies in the part of our brain that is our DMN (default mode network), which I think is what others may be referring to as the 'egoic' brain. The DMN focuses on past and future in order to provide solutions for survival; and this can be calmed by a different part of our brain which focuses on the present moment.

As the present moment is all there ever really is (everything else is just thoughts about past or future) then to spend most of our time using the latter part of our brain is much more beneficial to us on many levels, and mindfulness can help us to do this by reducing activity in the DMN . You can read more about this on the website of Dr Judson Brewer, a psychiatrist and cravings expert (http://www.judsonbrewer.com/).

Appendix 2

Summary of food and nutrients (briefly!)

Carbohydrates - from grains and starchy vegetables like potatoes – your body converts the starch to glucose, which is needed for energy and is essential for life. Simple carbohydrates, like bread and pasta, are converted to glucose quickly and so can cause a rapid increase in blood sugar levels. Other carbohydrates, like sweet potatoes, rice, legumes and root vegetables are absorbed much more slowly

Fats - from either animal products, or plants like avocados and nuts - your body converts the fat to essential fatty acids, which are needed for energy and to make hormones. These are essential fats that your body can't make and so need to be sourced from food; but should be eaten in moderation.

Proteins - from either animal products or from plants, including seeds and nuts – your body converts the amino acids gained from the proteins eaten, to human proteins which are needed for things like making hormones and repairing your body. Although each plant does not always have every amino acid that you need, if you eat a variety of vegetables you can get all the protein you need from a plant based diet.

Vitamins and minerals – you can get the ones you need by eating a variety of non-starchy vegetables, (which includes most vegetables other than potatoes), and fruits. They are needed for many things including energy, manufacture of hormones and general health.

Fibre – from vegetables and fruits. There are two kinds, non-soluble, which bulks out the food and helps in the process of moving it along the intestines which keeps them healthy; and soluble, which the commensal bacteria in the colon can digest and use as a food source. This, in turn, provides you with essential vitamins and other products like neurotransmitters.

Warning: If you eat an animal-free diet you can be deficient in vitamin B12 (cobalamin), which is found in animal products; but some seaweed, like nori (purple larva), is a fantastic source of vitamin B12, and you can also find it in yeast extract (like Marmite and Sainsburys Reduced Salt Yeast Extract). Any concerns can easily be resolved by taking a supplement of sublingual (dissolve under your tongue) methyl-cobalamin. The normal one you will see for sale is cyano-cobalamin, as this is cheaper to make, but your body needs the vitamin B12 with the methyl group rather than the cyanide (cyano) group!

FURTHER READING

The Autoimmune Solution by Amy Myers MD

Hashimoto's Thyroiditis: Lifestyle Interventions for Finding and Treating the Root Cause by Izabella Wentz

A New Earth by Eckhart Tolle

Practical Mindfulness by Ken A Verni Psy.D

Judson Brewer MD PhD; apps and website

Kris Carr – *Crazy Sexy Cancer*. http://kriscarr.com

References

Chapter One
1. Definition of Chronic disease. MedicineNet.com. Sourced March 9 2016
   http://www.medicinenet.com/script/main/art.asp?articlekey= 33490
2. Okada H, Kuhn C, Feillet H, Bach J-F. The "hygiene hypothesis" for autoimmune and allergic diseases: an update. Clinical and Experimental Immunology. 2010;160(1):1-9. doi:10.1111/j.1365-2249.2010.04139.x.

Chapter Two
3. Antibiotic Exposure by 6 Months and Asthma and Allergy at 6 Years: Findings in a Cohort of 1,401 US Children. Kari R. Risnes, Kathleen Belanger, William Murk and Michael B. Bracken. Oxford Journals Medicine & Health American Jnl of Epidemiology Volume 173, Issue 3Pp. 310-318.
4. The association of changes in physical-activity level and other lifestyle characteristics with mortality among men. Paffenbarger RS Jr, Hyde RT, Wing AL, Lee IM, Jung DL, Kampert JB. N Engl J Med. 1993 Feb 25;328(8):538-45.
5. Finishing the euchromatic sequence of the human genome. International Human Genome Sequencing Consortium. Nature 431, 931-945 (21 October 2004) | doi:10.1038/nature03001; Received 29 July 2004; Accepted 7 September 2004
6. The ENCODE Project Consortium. "A User's Guide to the Encyclopedia of DNA Elements (ENCODE)." Ed. Peter B. Becker. PLoS Biology 9.4 (2011): e1001046. PMC. Web. 4 Mar. 2016.
7. https://www.theguardian.com/science/blog/2011/sep/14/dark -matter-of-the-genome
8. The ENCODE Project Consortium. "A User's Guide to the Encyclopedia of DNA Elements (ENCODE)." Ed. Peter B. Becker. PLoS Biology 9.4 (2011): e1001046. PMC. Web. 4 Mar. 2016.

9. Morris, K.V., and J.S. Mattick. "The Rise of Regulatory RNA." Nature reviews. Genetics 15.6 (2014): 423–437. PMC. Web. 4 Mar. 2016.

10. Shammas, Masood A. "Telomeres, Lifestyle, Cancer, and Aging." Current Opinion in Clinical Nutrition and Metabolic Care 14.1 (2011): 28–34. PMC. Web. 4 Mar. 2016.

11. Junk DNA: A Journey Through the Dark Matter of the Genome. Nessa Carey

12. Shammas, Masood A. "Telomeres, Lifestyle, Cancer, and Aging." Current Opinion in Clinical Nutrition and Metabolic Care 14.1 (2011): 28–34. PMC. Web. 4 Mar. 2016.

13. Healthy lifestyle and leukocyte telomere length in U.S. women. Sun Q et al. PLoS One. 2012;7(5):e38374. doi: 10.1371/journal.pone.0038374. Epub 2012 May 31.

14. A meta-analytic review of the effects of mindfulness meditation on telomerase activity. Nicola S., John M. Malouff. Psychoneuroendocrinology April 2014Volume 42, Pages 45–48

15. Mindfulness-based cancer recovery and supportive-expressive therapy maintain telomere length relative to controls in distressed breast cancer survivors. Linda E. Carlson PhD et al. Cancer. Volume 121, Issue 3, pages 476–484, February 1, 2015

16. Dominguez-Salas, Paula et al. "DNA Methylation Potential: Dietary Intake and Blood Concentrations of One-Carbon Metabolites and Cofactors in Rural African Women." The American Journal of Clinical Nutrition 97.6 (2013): 1217–1227. PMC. Web. 4 Mar. 2016.

17. Epigenetic inheritance and evolution: A paternal perspective on dietary influences. Adelheid Soubry. Progress in Biophysics and Molecular Biology. Volume 118, Issues 1–2, July 2015, Pages 79–85. Epigenetic Inheritance and Programming.

18. Epigenetic inheritance and evolution: A paternal perspective on dietary influences. Adelheid Soubry. Progress in Biophysics and Molecular Biology. Volume 118, Issues 1–2, July 2015, Pages 79–85. Epigenetic Inheritance and Programming

19. Obesity at the age of 50 y in men and women exposed to famine prenatally. Anita CJ Ravelli *et al.* Am J Clin Nutr November 1999. vol. 70 no. 5 811-816.
20. Dominguez-Salas, Paula et al. "DNA Methylation Potential: Dietary Intake and Blood Concentrations of One-Carbon Metabolites and Cofactors in Rural African Women." The American Journal of Clinical Nutrition 97.6 (2013): 1217–1227. PMC. Web. 4 Mar. 2016.
21. Mother's Diet at Time of Conception May Alter Baby's DNA. Charles Q. Choi, Live Science Contributor. April 29, 2014 12:59pm ET
22. Dark matter of the genome. Nathan Green. The Guardian. Wednesday 14 September 2011 17.50 BST.
23. Galanin and galanin receptors in human cancers. Alexandra Berger *et al.* Neuropeptides. June 2005Volume 39, Issue 3, Pages 353–359.
24. Galanin and its receptors in neurological disorders. Linda Lundström *et al.* NeuroMolecular Medicine. January 2005, Volume 7, Issue 1, pp 157-180.
25. Epigenetics: genes, environment and the generation game. Angela Saini. The Observer. Sunday 7 September 2014 00.04 BST
26. Methylomic analysis of monozygotic twins discordant for autism spectrum disorder and related behavioural traits. C C Y Wong *et al.* Molecular Psychiatry (2014) 19, 495–503; doi:10.1038/mp.2013.41;published online 23 April 2013.
27. Methylomic analysis of monozygotic twins discordant for autism spectrum disorder and related behavioural traits. C C Y Wong et al. Molecular Psychiatry (2014) 19, 495–503; doi:10.1038/mp.2013.41;published online 23 April 2013.
28. DNA Methylation Signatures Triggered by Prenatal Maternal Stress Exposure to a Natural Disaster: Project Ice Storm. Lei Cao-Lei *et al.* September 19, 2014DOI: 10.1371/journal.pone.0107653
29. HLA gene family. U.S. National Library of medicine, online. Published: February 29, 2016
30. HLA gene family. U.S. National Library of medicine, online. Published: February 29, 2016

Chapter Three

31. https://www.nlm.nih.gov/medlineplus/ency/article/002222.htm
32. Chapter 6, Proteins and Amino Acids; online pdf http://awbc.com/info/blake/assets/pdf/Salge_Nutrition_Ch06.pdf
33. Histology and Cell Biology: An Introduction to Pathology. 11 Apr 2011by Abraham L Kierszenbaum M.D. Ph.D., Laura Tres M.D. Ph.D. (book)
34. Intestinal Barrier Function: Molecular Regulation and Disease Pathogenesis; Katherine R. Groschwitz, BS and Simon P. Hogan, PhD. J Allergy Clin Immunol. Author manuscript; available in PMC 2014 Dec 16. Published in final edited form as: J Allergy Clin Immunol. 2009 Jul; 124(1): 3–22. doi: 10.1016/j.jaci.2009.05.038

Chapter Four

35. Why Your Immune System Doesn't Eat You Alive; Esther Landhuis; Scientific American, May 21, 2015
36. Helper T Cells and Lymphocyte Activation; Molecular Biology of the Cell. 4th edition. Garland Science, 2002.
37. Zhang, Jun-Ming, and Jianxiong An. "Cytokines, Inflammation and Pain." International anesthesiology clinics 45.2 (2007): 27–37. PMC. Web. 8 Mar. 2016.
38. The Association of changes in Physical Activity Level and Other Lifestyle Characteristics with Mortality among Men. Ralph Paffenbarger, Jnr., MD. The new England Journal of Medicine. Feb 25, 1993.

Chapter Five

39. That gut feeling, review by Dr. Siri Carpenter. American Psychological Association, September 2012, Vol 43, No. 8.
40. Glycans in the immune system and The Altered Glycan Theory of Autoimmunity: A critical review Emanual Maverakisa, Kyoungmi Kimb, Michiko Shimodaa, M. Eric Gershwinc, Forum Patela, Reason Wilkena, Siba Raychaudhuric, L. Renee Ruhaakb, Carlito B. Lebrillad, Journal of Autoimmunity, Volume 57, February 2015, Pages 1–13

41. Essentials of Glycobiology. 2nd edition. Varki A, Cummings RD, Esko JD, et al., editors. Cold Spring Harbor (NY): Cold Spring Harbor Laboratory Press; 2009. Chapter Six

42. Commensal Bacteria and Epithelial Cross Talk in the Developing Intestine. Samuli Rautava, MD, PhD and W. Allan Walker, MD. Curr Gastroenterol Rep. 2007 Oct; 9(5): 385–392.

43. Hooper LV. Bacterial contributions to mammalian gut development. Trends Microbiol. 2004;12:129–134. [PubMed]

44. Epigenetic Control of the Host Gene by Commensal Bacteria in Large Intestinal Epithelial Cells. Kyoko Takahashi1, Yutaka Sugi, Kou Nakano, Masato Tsuda, Kenta Kurihara, Akira Hosono and Shuichi Kaminogawa . October 14, 2011, The Journal of Biological Chemistry, 286, 35755-35762. http://www.jbc.org/content/286/41/35755.full

45. Epigenetic Control of the Host Gene by Commensal Bacteria in Large Intestinal Epithelial Cells. Kyoko Takahashi1, Yutaka Sugi, Kou Nakano, Masato Tsuda, Kenta Kurihara, Akira Hosono and Shuichi Kaminogawa . October 14, 2011, The Journal of Biological Chemistry, 286, 35755-35762. http://www.jbc.org/content/286/41/35755.full

Chapter Six

46. Recognition of Commensal Microflora by Toll-Like Receptors Is Required for Intestinal Homeostasis. Seth Rakoff-Nahoum1, Justin Paglino2, Fatima Eslami-Varzaneh3, Stephen Edberg2, Ruslan Medzhitov. Science Direct. Volume 118, Issue 2, 23 July 2004, Pages 229–241

47. Recognition of commensal microflora by toll-like receptors is required for intestinal homeostasis. Rakoff-Nahoum S, Paglino J, Eslami-Varzaneh F, Edberg S, Medzhitov R. Cell. 2004 Jul 23;118(2):229-41.

48. Backhed F, Ley RE, SonnenburgJL, Peterson DA, Gordon JI. Host-bacterial mutualism in the human intestine. Science 2005;307:1915–20.

49. Hooper LV, WongMH, Thelin A, Hansson L, Falk PG, Gordon JI. Molecular analysis of commensal host-microbial relationships in the intestine. Science 2001;291:881–4.

50. SonnenburgJL, Xu J, Leip DD, Chen CH, Westover BP, Weatherford J, Buhler JD, Gordon JI. Glycan foraging in vivo by an intestine-adapted bacterial symbiont. Science 2005; 307:1955–9.

51. Wostmann BS, Larkin C, Moriarty A, Bruckner-Kardoss E. Dietary intake, energy metabolism, and excretory losses of adult male germfree Wistar rats. Lab Anim Sci 1983; 33:46–50

52. Den Besten, Gijs et al. The Role of Short-Chain Fatty Acids in the Interplay between Diet, Gut Microbiota, and Host Energy Metabolism. Journal of Lipid Research 54.9 (2013): 2325–2340. PMC. Web. 31 July 2015. Sourced online at http://www.ncbi.nlm.nih.gov/pmc/articles/PMC3735932/#!p o=1.13636

53. Binder HJ1. Role of colonic short-chain fatty acid transport in diarrhea. Annu Rev Physiol. 2010; 72:297-313. doi: 10.1146/annurev-physiol-021909-135817.

54. Butyrate enhances the intestinal barrier by facilitating tight junction assembly via activation of AMP-activated protein kinase in Caco-2 cell monolayers. Peng L1, Li ZR, Green RS, Holzman IR, Lin J. J Nutr. 2009 Sep;139(9):1619-25. doi: 10.3945/jn.109.104638. Epub 2009 Jul 22.

55. Bacteria as vitamin suppliers to their host: a gut microbiota perspective. LeBlanc JG et al; Curr Opin Biotechnol. 2013 Apr;24(2):160-8. doi: 10.1016/j.copbio.2012.08.005. Epub 2012 Aug 30.

56. The production of menaquinones (vitamin K2) by intestinal bacteria and their role in maintaining coagulation homeostasis. Conly JM, Stein K. Prog Food Nutr Sci. 1992 Oct-Dec;16(4):307-43.

57. Human nutrition, the gut microbiome, and immune system: envisioning the future. Kau, Andrew L. et al. Nature 474.7351 (2011): 327–336. PMC. Web. 8 Mar. 2016.

58. Pharmacometabonomic identification of a significant host-microbiome metabolic interaction affecting human drug metabolism. T. Andrew Clayton, David Baker, John C. Lindon, Jeremy R. Everett, and Jeremy K. Nicholsona. Proc Natl Acad Sci U S A. 2009 Aug 25; 106(34): 14728–14733. Published online 2009 Aug 10. doi: 10.1073/pnas.0904489106 http://www.ncbi.nlm.nih.gov/pmc/articles/PMC2731842/

59. Gut microbes important for serotonin production. Catharine Paddock PhD, 21 April 2015. Medical News Today. http://www.medicalnewstoday.com/articles/292693.php

60. Indigenous Bacteria from the Gut Microbiota Regulate Host Serotonin Biosynthesis. Jessica M. Yano et al., 2015, Cell 161, 264–276 April 9, 2015

61. Gut microbes important for serotonin production. Catharine Paddock PhD, 21 April 2015. Medical News Today. http://www.medicalnewstoday.com/articles/292693.php

62. http://en.m.wikipedia.org/wiki/Gut_flora

63. Pharmacometabonomic identification of a significant host-microbiome metabolic interaction affecting human drug metabolism. T. Andrew Clayton, David Baker, John C. Lindon, Jeremy R. Everett, and Jeremy K. Nicholsona. Proc Natl Acad Sci U S A. 2009 Aug 25; 106(34): 14728–14733. Published online 2009 Aug 10. doi: 10.1073/pnas.0904489106 http://www.ncbi.nlm.nih.gov/pmc/articles/PMC2731842/

64. Pharmacometabonomic identification of a significant host-microbiome metabolic interaction affecting human drug metabolism. T. Andrew Clayton, David Baker, John C. Lindon, Jeremy R. Everett, and Jeremy K. Nicholsona. Proc Natl Acad Sci U S A. 2009 Aug 25; 106(34): 14728–14733. Published online 2009 Aug 10. doi: 10.1073/pnas.0904489106 http://www.ncbi.nlm.nih.gov/pmc/articles/PMC2731842/

65. From Human Genetics and Genomics to Pharmacogenetics and Pharmacogenomics: Past Lessons, Future Directions. Daniel W. Nebert, Ge Zhang, and Elliot S. Vesell. Drug Metab Rev. Author manuscript; available in PMC 2009 Sep 26. Published in final edited form as: Drug Metab Rev. 2008; 40(2): 187–224. doi: 10.1080/03602530801952864. http://www.ncbi.nlm.nih.gov/pmc/articles/PMC2752627/

66. Pharmaco-metabonomic phenotyping and personalized drug treatment. Clayton TA et al., Nature. 2006 Apr 20;440(7087):1073-7.

67. Miller, A. W., & Dearing, D. (2013). The Metabolic and Ecological Interactions of Oxalate-Degrading Bacteria in the Mammalian Gut. Pathogens, 2(4), 636–652. http://doi.org/10.3390/pathogens2040636

68. Drug metabolism: manipulating the microbiome. The Pharmaceutical Journal 27 MAR 2015 By Sarah DeWeerdt

69. Host-microbial interactions in the metabolism of therapeutic and diet-derived xenobiotics. Rachel N. Carmody, Peter J. Turnbaugh. J Clin Invest. 2014;124(10):4173-4181. doi:10.1172/JCI72335.

70. Probiotic gut effect prevents the chronic psychological stress-induced brain activity abnormality in mice. A. AIT-BELGNAOUI et al., Neurogastroenterol Motil (2014) 26, 510–520.

71. Regulation of spontaneous intestinal tumorigenesis through the adaptor protein MyD88. Rakoff-Nahoum S1, Medzhitov R. Science. 2007 Jul 6;317(5834):124-7.

72. Induction of colonic regulatory T cells by indigenous Clostridium species. Atarashi K et al., Science. 2011 Jan 21;331(6015):337-41. doi: 10.1126/science.1198469. Epub 2010 Dec 23.

73. Round, J. L., & Mazmanian, S. K. (2009). The gut microbiome shapes intestinal immune responses during health and disease. Nature Reviews. Immunology, 9(5), 313–323. http://doi.org/10.1038/nri2515

Chapter Seven

74. Albenberg, L. G., & Wu, G. D. (2014). Diet and the Intestinal Microbiome: Associations, Functions, and Implications for Health and Disease. Gastroenterology, 146(6), 1564–1572. http://doi.org/10.1053/j.gastro.2014.01.058

75. Whitman, W. B., Coleman, D. C., & Wiebe, W. J. (1998). Prokaryotes: The unseen majority. Proceedings of the National Academy of Sciences of the United States of America, 95(12), 6578–6583.

76. An obesity-associated gut microbiome with increased capacity for energy harvest. Turnbaugh PJ *et al.,* Nature. 2006 Dec 21;444(7122):1027-31.

77. Eckburg, P. B., Bik, E. M., Bernstein, C. N., Purdom, E., Dethlefsen, L., Sargent, M., ... Relman, D. A. (2005). Diversity of the Human Intestinal Microbial Flora. Science (New York, N.Y.), 308(5728), 1635–1638. http://doi.org/10.1126/science.1110591

78. Frank, D. N., St. Amand, A. L., Feldman, R. A., Boedeker, E. C., Harpaz, N., & Pace, N. R. (2007). Molecular-phylogenetic characterization of microbial community imbalances in human inflammatory bowel diseases. Proceedings of the National Academy of Sciences of the United States of America, 104(34), 13780–13785. http://doi.org/10.1073/pnas.0706625104

79. Extending Our View of Self: the Human Gut Microbiome Initiative (HGMI). Jeffrey I. Gordon *et al.,* http://www.genome.gov/pages/research/sequencing/seqprop osals/hgmiseq.pdf

80. γ-Aminobutyric acid production by culturable bacteria from the human intestine. Barrett E *et al.,* J Appl Microbiol. 2012 Aug;113(2):411-7. doi: 10.1111/j.1365-2672.2012.05344.x. Epub 2012 Jun 15.

81. A randomized controlled trial to test the effect of multispecies probiotics on cognitive reactivity to sad mood. Steenbergen L *et al.,* Brain Behav Immun. 2015 Aug;48:258-64. doi: 10.1016/j.bbi.2015.04.003. Epub 2015 Apr 7.

82. Drugs and Supplements. Acidophilus (Lactobacillus acidophilus). Mayo Clinic http://www.mayoclinic.org/drugs-supplements/acidophilus/background/hrb-20058615

83. Lee, B. J., & Bak, Y.-T. (2011). Irritable Bowel Syndrome, Gut Microbiota and Probiotics. Journal of Neurogastroenterology and Motility, 17(3), 252–266. http://doi.org/10.5056/jnm.2011.17.3.252

84. Ingestion of Lactobacillus strain regulates emotional behavior and central GABA receptor expression in a mouse via the vagus nerve. Bravo JA, et al., Proc Natl Acad Sci U S A. 2011 Sep 20;108(38):16050-5. doi: 10.1073/pnas.1102999108. Epub 2011 Aug 29.

85. γ-Aminobutyric acid production by culturable bacteria from the human intestine. Barrett E et al., J Appl Microbiol. 2012 Aug;113(2):411-7. doi: 10.1111/j.1365-2672.2012.05344.x. Epub 2012 Jun 15.

86. Probiotic gut effect prevents the chronic psychological stress-induced brain activity abnormality in mice. A. Ait-Belgnaoui et al., Neurogastroenterology & Motility. Volume 26, Issue 4, pages 510–520, April 2014

87. Lactobacillus rossiae, a Vitamin B12 Producer, Represents a Metabolically Versatile Species within the Genus Lactobacillus. Maria De Angelis et al., Plos.org., September 29, 2014DOI: 10.1371/journal.pone.0107232

88. Lactobacillus rossiae, a Vitamin B12 Producer, Represents a Metabolically Versatile Species within the Genus Lactobacillus. Maria De Angelis et al., Plos.org., September 29, 2014DOI: 10.1371/journal.pone.0107232

89. Lactobacillus plantarum as a Strategy for an In situ production of Vitamin B2. Mattia Pia Arenal et al., J Food Nutr Disor 2014, S1 http://dx.doi.org/10.4172/2324-9323.S1-004

90. Bacteroides dorei dominates gut microbiome prior to autoimmunity in Finnish children at high risk for type 1 diabetes. Austin G. Davis-Richardson et al., Front. Microbiol., 10 December 2014 | http://dx.doi.org/10.3389/fmicb.2014.00678.

91. The association between autism and errors in early embryogenesis: what is the causal mechanism? Ploeger A *et al.*, Biol Psychiatry. 2010 Apr 1;67(7):602-7. doi: 10.1016/j.biopsych.2009.10.010. Epub 2009 Nov 22.
92. Wu, T., Zhang, Z., Liu, B., Hou, D., Liang, Y., Zhang, J., & Shi, P. (2013). Gut microbiota dysbiosis and bacterial community assembly associated with cholesterol gallstones in large-scale study. BMC Genomics, 14, 669. http://doi.org/10.1186/1471-2164-14-669
93. Bhattacharjee, S., & Lukiw, W. J. (2013). Alzheimer's disease and the microbiome. Frontiers in Cellular Neuroscience, 7, 153. http://doi.org/10.3389/fncel.2013.00153
94. Genomic Insights into Bifidobacteria. Ju-Hoon Lee and Daniel J. O'Sullivan. doi: 10.1128/MMBR.00004-10 Microbiol. Mol. Biol. Rev. September 2010 vol. 74 no. 3 378-416 1 September 2010
95. Human milk oligosaccharides are resistant to enzymatic hydrolysis in the upper gastrointestinal tract. Engfer MB *et al.*, Am J Clin Nutr. 2000 Jun;71(6):1589-96.
96. Human milk oligosaccharides are resistant to enzymatic hydrolysis in the upper gastrointestinal tract. Engfer MB et al., Am J Clin Nutr. 2000 Jun;71(6):1589-96.
97. Probiotics and Prebiotics: where are we going? Chapter Four. Takahiro Matsuki *et al.*, Edited by Gerald W Tannock.
98. Probiotic gut effect prevents the chronic psychological stress-induced brain activity abnormality in mice. A. Ait-Belgnaoui *et al.*, Neurogastroenterology & Motility. Volume 26, Issue 4, pages 510–520, April 2014.
99. Fungal Signature in the Gut Microbiota of Pediatric Patients with Inflammatory Bowel Disease. Chehoud C, *et al.*, Inflamm Bowel Dis. 2015 Aug;21(8):1948-56. doi: 10.1097/MIB.0000000000000454.
100. The emerging world of the fungal microbiome. Gary B. Huffnagle, Mairi C. Noverr. Trends in Microbiology. Volume 21, Issue 7, July 2013, Pages 334–341.

101. White, S. J., Rosenbach, A., Lephart, P., Nguyen, D., Benjamin, A., Tzipori, S., ... Kumamoto, C. A. (2007). Self-Regulation of Candida albicans Population Size during GI Colonization. PLoS Pathogens, 3(12), e184. http://doi.org/10.1371/journal.ppat.0030184

102. Striking a Balance: Fungal Commensalism versus Pathogenesis. Iliyan D. Iliev, David M. Underhill. Curr Opin Microbiol. 2013 Jun; 16(3): 366–373. http://www.ncbi.nlm.nih.gov/pmc/articles/PMC3742553 Published online 2013 Jun 4. doi: 10.1016/j.mib.2013.05.004

Chapter Eight

103. http://ghr.nlm.nih.gov/geneFamily/hla

104. http://ghr.nlm.nih.gov/geneFamily/hla

105. Microbial ecology: human gut microbes associated with obesity. Ley RE et al., Nature. 2006 Dec 21;444(7122):1022-3.

106. An obesity-associated gut microbiome with increased capacity for energy harvest.. Turnbaugh PJ et al., Nature. 2006 Dec 21;444(7122):1027-31.

107. Muegge, B. D., Kuczynski, J., Knights, D., Clemente, J. C., González, A., Fontana, L., ... Gordon, J. I. (2011). Diet drives convergence in gut microbiome functions across mammalian phylogeny and within humans. Science (New York, N.y.), 332(6032), 970–974. http://doi.org/10.1126/science.1198719

108. The Firmicutes/Bacteroidetes ratio of the human microbiota changes with age. Mariat D et al., BMC Microbiol. 2009 Jun 9;9:123. doi: 10.1186/1471-2180-9-123.

109. Cruchet, S., Furnes, R., Maruy, A., Hebel, E., Palacios, J., Medina, F., ... Zablah, R. A. (2015). The Use of Probiotics in Pediatric Gastroenterology: A Review of the Literature and Recommendations by Latin-American Experts. Paediatric Drugs, 17(3), 199–216. http://doi.org/10.1007/s40272-015-0124-6

110. Critical review: vegetables and fruit in the prevention of chronic diseases. Eur J Nutr. 2012 Sep; 51(6): 637–663. Published online 2012 Jun 9. doi: 10.1007/s00394-012-0380-y. Heiner Boeing, Angela Bechthold,corresponding author Achim Bub, Sabine Ellinger, Dirk Haller, Anja Kroke, Eva Leschik-Bonnet, Manfred J. Müller, Helmut Oberritter, Matthias Schulze, Peter Stehle, and Bernhard Watzl

111. The effect of diet on the human gut microbiome: a metagenomic analysis in humanized gnotobiotic mice. Turnbaugh PJ et al., Sci Transl Med. 2009 Nov 11;1(6):6ra14. doi: 10.1126/scitranslmed.3000322.

112. Whole Grains, Legumes, and the Subsequent Meal Effect: Implications for Blood Glucose Control and the Role of Fermentation. Janine A. Higgins. J Nutr Mctab. 2012; 2012: 829238. Published online 2011 Oct 30. doi: 10.1155/2012/829238.

113. Higgins, J. A. (2012). Whole Grains, Legumes, and the Subsequent Meal Effect: Implications for Blood Glucose Control and the Role of Fermentation. Journal of Nutrition and Metabolism, 2012, 829238. http://doi.org/10.1155/2012/829238

114. Effects of Dietary Fiber and Carbohydrate on Glucose and Lipoprotein Metabolism in Diabetic Patients. Gabriele Riccardi, MD and Angela A Rivellese, MD. doi: 10.2337/diacare.14.12.1115 Diabetes Care December 1991 vol. 14 no. 12 1115-1125.

115. A Soluble Fiber Primer — Plus the Top Five Foods That Can Lower LDL Cholesterol. By Judith C. Thalheimer, RD, LDN. Today's Dietitian Vol. 15 No. 12 P. 16

116. Savignac HM, Corona G, Mills H, et al. Prebiotic feeding elevates central brain derived neurotrophic factor, N-methyl-d-aspartate receptor subunits and d-serine. Neurochemistry International. 2013;63(8):756-764. doi:10.1016/j.neuint.2013.10.006.

117. Personalized Nutrition by Prediction of Glycemic Responses. David Zeevi et al., Cell, Volume 163, Issue 5, p1079–1094, 19 November 2015.

118. Personalized Nutrition by Prediction of Glycemic Responses. David Zeevi et al., Cell, Volume 163, Issue 5, p1079–1094, 19 November 2015.

119. Lactobacillus brevis OK56 ameliorates high-fat diet-induced obesity in mice by inhibiting NF-κB activation and gut microbial LPS production. Kyung-Ah Kim et al., Journal of Functional Foods, Volume 13, March 2015, Pages 183–191.

Chapter Nine

120. Celiac Disease, Terry L. Smith. The Rosen Publishing Group, 1 Sep 2006

121. Willem-Karel Dicke: Pioneer in Gluten-free Diet in the Treatment of Celiac Disease. By Jefferson Adams Celiac.com. Published 05/14/2010.

122. Infections of the Gastrointestinal System. Chetana Vaishnavi. JP Medical Ltd, 31 Mar 2013

123. RHR: Pioneering Researcher Alessio Fasano M.D. on Gluten, Autoimmunity & Leaky Gut. Published AUGUST 8, 2012 by CHRIS KRESSER. http://chriskresser.com/pioneering-researcher-alessio-fasano-m-d-on-gluten-autoimmunity-leaky-gut/

124. Klöck C, DiRaimondo TR, Khosla C. Role of Transglutaminase 2 in Celiac Disease Pathogenesis. Seminars in immunopathology. 2012;34(4):513-522. doi:10.1007/s00281-012-0305-0.

125. Fasano A. Zonulin, regulation of tight junctions, and autoimmune diseases. Annals of the New York Academy of Sciences. 2012;1258(1):25-33. doi:10.1111/j.1749-6632.2012.06538.x.

126. Zonulin, a newly discovered modulator of intestinal permeability, and its expression in coeliac disease. Fasano A et al., Lancet. 2000 Apr 29;355(9214):1518-9.

127. Zonulin and Its Regulation of Intestinal Barrier Function: The Biological Door to Inflammation, Autoimmunity, and Cancer. Alessio Fasano. Physiological Reviews Published 1 January 2011 Vol. 91 no. 1, 151-175 DOI: 10.1152/physrev.00003.2008

128. Bethune MT, Khosla C. Parallels between Pathogens and Gluten Peptides in Celiac Sprue. Finlay BB, ed. PLoS Pathogens. 2008;4(2):e34. doi:10.1371/journal.ppat.0040034.

129. Groschwitz KR, Hogan SP. Intestinal Barrier Function: Molecular Regulation and Disease Pathogenesis. The Journal of allergy and clinical immunology. 2009;124(1):3-22. doi:10.1016/j.jaci.2009.05.038.

130. Tripathi A, Lammers KM, Goldblum S, et al. Identification of human zonulin, a physiological modulator of tight junctions, as prehaptoglobin-2. Proceedings of the National Academy of Sciences of the United States of America. 2009;106(39):16799-16804. doi:10.1073/pnas.0906773106.

131. Zonulin and Its Regulation of Intestinal Barrier Function: The Biological Door to Inflammation, Autoimmunity, and Cancer. Alessio Fasano. Physiological Reviews Published 1 January 2011 Vol. 91 no. 1, 151-175 DOI: 10.1152/physrev.00003.2008.

132. Intestinal digestive resistance of immunodominant gliadin peptides. Hausch F et al., Am J Physiol Gastrointest Liver Physiol. 2002 Oct;283(4):G996-G1003.

133. Bethune MT, Khosla C. Parallels between Pathogens and Gluten Peptides in Celiac Sprue. Finlay BB, ed. PLoS Pathogens. 2008;4(2):e34. doi:10.1371/journal.ppat.0040034.

134. Zonulin and Its Regulation of Intestinal Barrier Function: The Biological Door to Inflammation, Autoimmunity, and Cancer. Alessio Fasano. Physiological Reviews Published 1 January 2011 Vol. 91 no. 1, 151-175 DOI: 10.1152/physrev.00003.2008

135. Hewagama A, Richardson B. The genetics and epigenetics of autoimmune diseases. Journal of autoimmunity. 2009;33(1):3. doi:10.1016/j.jaut.2009.03.007.

136. Hewagama A, Richardson B. The genetics and epigenetics of autoimmune diseases. Journal of autoimmunity. 2009;33(1):3. doi:10.1016/j.jaut.2009.03.007.

137. Leaky gut and autoimmune diseases. Fasano A. Clin Rev Allergy Immunol. 2012 Feb;42(1):71-8. doi: 10.1007/s12016-011-8291-x.

138. Increased gastrointestinal permeability is an early lesion in the spontaneously diabetic BB rat. J. B. Meddings *et al.*, American Journal of Physiology - Gastrointestinal and Liver Physiology Published 1 April 1999 Vol. 276 no. 4, G951-G957 DOI:

139. Intestinal permeability is increased in bronchial asthma. Z Hijazi *et al.*, Arch Dis Child 2004;89:227-229 doi:10.1136/adc.2003.027680

140. The blood-brain-barrier in multiple sclerosis: functional roles and therapeutic targeting. Correale J *et al.*, Autoimmunity. 2007 Mar;40(2):148-60.

141. Skardelly M, Armbruster FP, Meixensberger J, Hilbig H. Expression of Zonulin, c-kit, and Glial Fibrillary Acidic Protein in Human Gliomas. Translational Oncology. 2009;2(3):117-120.

142. Skardelly M, Armbruster FP, Mcixensberger J, Hilbig H. Expression of Zonulin, c-kit, and Glial Fibrillary Acidic Protein in Human Gliomas. Translational Oncology. 2009;2(3):117-120.

143. Dysbiosis of the gut microbiota in disease. Simon Carding *et al.*, Microbial Ecology in Health and Disease. Home > Vol 26 (2015) >Carding

144. Dysbiosis of the gut microbiota in disease. Simon Carding *et al.*, Microbial Ecology in Health and Disease. Home > Vol 26 (2015) >Carding

145. Tripathi A, Lammers KM, Goldblum S, et al. Identification of human zonulin, a physiological modulator of tight junctions, as prehaptoglobin-2. Proceedings of the National Academy of Sciences of the United States of America. 2009;106(39):16799-16804. doi:10.1073/pnas.0906773106.

146. Leaky gut and autoimmune diseases. Fasano A. Clin Rev Allergy Immunol. 2012 Feb;42(1):71-8. doi: 10.1007/s12016-011-8291-x.

147. Molecular mimicry as a mechanism for food immune reactivities and autoimmunity. Vojdani A. Altern Ther Health Med. 2015;21 Suppl 1:34-45.

148. Molecular mimicry as a mechanism for food immune reactivities and autoimmunity. Vojdani A. Altern Ther Health Med. 2015;21 Suppl 1:34-45.
149. Molecular mimicry as a mechanism for food immune reactivities and autoimmunity. Vojdani A. Altern Ther Health Med. 2015;21 Suppl 1:34-45.
150. Molecular mimicry as a mechanism for food immune reactivities and autoimmunity. Vojdani A. Altern Ther Health Med. 2015;21 Suppl 1:34-45.
151. Cusick MF, Libbey JE, Fujinami RS. Molecular Mimicry as a Mechanism of Autoimmune Disease. Clinical reviews in allergy & immunology. 2012;42(1):102-111. doi:10.1007/s12016-011-8294-7.
152. The Prevalence of Antibodies against Wheat and Milk Proteins in Blood Donors and Their Contribution to Neuroimmune Reactivities. Aristo Vojdani *et al.*, Nutrients 2014, 6(1), 15-36; doi:10.3390/nu6010015
153. The Prevalence of Antibodies against Wheat and Milk Proteins in Blood Donors and Their Contribution to Neuroimmune Reactivities. Aristo Vojdani. Nutrients 2014, 6(1), 15-36; doi:10.3390/nu6010015
154. Food toxins, molecular mimicry, leaky gut and the MS connection by Lynn Toohey, Ph.D. listed in cellular chemistry, originally published in issue 18 - March 1997 http://www.positivehealth.com/article/cellular-chemistry/food-toxins-molecular-mimicry-leaky-gut-and-the-ms-connection
155. Leaky Gut Syndrome in Plain English – and How to Fix It by JORDAN REASONER. http://scdlifestyle.com/2010/03/the-scd-diet-and-leaky-gut-syndrome/
156. Leaky Gut Syndrome in Plain English – and How to Fix It by JORDAN REASONER. http://scdlifestyle.com/2010/03/the-scd-diet-and-leaky-gut-syndrome/
157. Leaky Gut Syndrome in Plain English – and How to Fix It by JORDAN REASONER. http://scdlifestyle.com/2010/03/the-scd-diet-and-leaky-gut-syndrome/

158. Leaky Gut Syndrome in Plain English – and How to Fix It by JORDAN REASONER. http://scdlifestyle.com/2010/03/the-scd-diet-and-leaky-gut-syndrome/

159. Leaky Gut Syndrome in Plain English – and How to Fix It by JORDAN REASONER. http://scdlifestyle.com/2010/03/the-scd-diet-and-leaky-gut-syndrome/

160. Rubio-Tapia A, Kyle RA, Kaplan EL, et al. Increased Prevalence and Mortality in Undiagnosed Celiac Disease. Gastroenterology. 2009;137(1):88-93. doi:10.1053/j.gastro.2009.03.059.

161. Fasano A. Zonulin, regulation of tight junctions, and autoimmune diseases. Annals of the New York Academy of Sciences. 2012;1258(1):25-33. doi:10.1111/j.1749-6632.2012.06538.x.

162. The Gluten Effect: How "Innocent" Wheat Is Ruining Your Health Paperback – 13 Feb 2009 by Dr Vikki Petersen

163. Hill JM, Bhattacharjee S, Pogue AI, Lukiw WJ. The Gastrointestinal Tract Microbiome and Potential Link to Alzheimer's Disease. Frontiers in Neurology. 2014;5:43. doi:10.3389/fneur.2014.00043.

164. New understanding of gluten sensitivity. Volta U; De Giorgio R. Nat Rev Gastroenterol Hepatol. 2012 Feb 28;9(5):295-9. doi: 10.1038/nrgastro.2012.15.

165. Effect of gluten free diet on immune response to gliadin in patients with non-celiac gluten sensitivity. Giacomo Caio et al., BMC Gastroenterology201414:26 DOI: 10.1186/1471-230X-14-26© Caio et al.; licensee BioMed Central Ltd. 2014 Received: 9 November 2013 Accepted: 5 February 2014 Published: 13 February 2014

166. Aluminum and Glyphosate Can Synergistically Induce Pineal Gland Pathology: Connection to Gut Dysbiosis and Neurological DiseaseStephanie Seneff1, Nancy Swanson2, Chen Li1. Agricultural Sciences, Vol.06 No.01(2015), Article ID:53106,28 pages 10.4236/as.2015.61005

167. Aluminum and Glyphosate Can Synergistically Induce Pineal Gland Pathology: Connection to Gut Dysbiosis and Neurological DiseaseStephanie Seneff1, Nancy Swanson2, Chen Li1. Agricultural Sciences, Vol.06 No.01(2015), Article ID:53106,28 pages 10.4236/as.2015.61005

168. Glyphosate, pathways to modern diseases II: Celiac sprue and gluten intolerance. Anthony Samsel1 and Stephanie SeneffL1. Interdiscip Toxicol. 2013 Dec; 6(4): 159–184. Published online 2013 Dec. doi: 10.2478/intox-2013-0026

169. Yokote H, Miyake S, Croxford JL, Oki S, Mizusawa H, Yamamura T. NKT Cell-Dependent Amelioration of a Mouse Model of Multiple Sclerosis by Altering Gut Flora. The American Journal of Pathology. 2008;173(6):1714-1723. doi:10.2353/ajpath.2008.080622.

170. Commensal Gut Bacteria and the Etiopathogenesis of Rheumatoid Arthritis. CHRISTOPHER J. EDWARDS. J Rheumatol 2008;35;1477-1479

171. Inflammatory bowel disease: the role of environmental factors. Danese S1; Sans M, Fiocchi C. Autoimmun Rev. 2004 Jul;3(5):394-400.

172. Diabetes-Specific HLA-DR–Restricted Proinflammatory T-Cell Response to Wheat Polypeptides in Tissue Transglutaminase Antibody–Negative Patients With Type 1 Diabetes. Majid Mojibian et al., Diabetes August 2009 vol. 58 no. 8 1789-1796

173. Simpson M, Mojibian M, Barriga K, et al. An exploration of Glb1 Homologue AntibodyLevels in Children at Increased Risk for Type 1 Diabetes mellitus. Pediatric diabetes. 2009;10(8):563. doi:10.1111/j.1399-5448.2009.00541.x.

174. Is it dietary insulin? Vaarala O. Ann N Y Acad Sci. 2006 Oct;1079:350-9.

175. Doctor in the House, BBC1: Dr Rangan Chatterjee implements a strict health regime on a London family in new documentary. Evening Standard. Thursday 19 November 2015

Chapter Ten
176. Anatomy and physiology of the enteric nervous system. M Costa, S J H Brookes, G W Hennig. Chapter 2. Gut 2000;47:iv15-iv19 doi:10.1136/gut.47.suppl_4.iv15
177. The Enteric Nervous System: The Brain in the Gut. http://www.psyking.net/id36.htm
178. Serotonin, tryptophan metabolism and the brain-gut-microbiome axis. S.M. O'Mahony *et al.*, Behavioural Brain Research, Volume 277, 15 January 2015, Pages 32–48
179. Savignac HM, Corona G, Mills H, et al. Prebiotic feeding elevates central brain derived neurotrophic factor, N-methyl-d-aspartate receptor subunits and d-serine. Neurochemistry International. 2013;63(8):756-764. doi:10.1016/j.neuint.2013.10.006.
180. Immunomodulatory Effects of Probiotics in the Intestinal Tract. V. Delcenserie *et al., Curr. Issues Mol. Biol. 10: 37-54.*
181. Ingestion of Lactobacillus strain regulates emotional behavior and central GABA receptor expression in a mouse via the vagus nerve. Bravo J. et al., vol. 108 no. 38. 16050–16055 http://m.pnas.org/content/108/38/16050.full
182. Administration of Lactobacillus helveticus NS8 improves behavioral, cognitive, and biochemical aberrations caused by chronic restraint stress. Liang S *et al.,* Neuroscience. 2015 Dec 3;310:561-77. doi: 10.1016/j.neuroscience.2015.09.033. Epub 2015 Sep 25
183. Ingestion of Lactobacillus strain regulates emotional behavior and central GABA receptor expression in a mouse via the vagus nerve. Bravo J. et al., vol. 108 no. 38. 16050–16055 http://m.pnas.org/content/108/38/16050.full
184. Passage of cytokines across the blood-brain barrier. Banks WA *et al., Neuroimmunomodulation. 1995 Jul-Aug;2(4):241-8.*
185. Tillisch K. The effects of gut microbiota on CNS function in humans. Gut Microbes. 2014;5(3):404-410. doi:10.4161/gmic.29232.

186. Probiotic treatment of rat pups normalises corticosterone release and ameliorates colonic dysfunction induced by maternal separation. Gareau MG *et al.*, Gut. 2007 Nov;56(11):1522-8. Epub 2007 Mar 5.
187. The neurobiology of stress and gastrointestinal disease. Review. E. Mayer. Gut 2000;47:861–869
188. Effects of stressful life events on bowel symptoms: subjects with irritable bowel syndrome compared with subjects without bowel dysfunction. Whitehead WE, Crowell MD, Robinson JC, Heller BR, Schuster MM. Gut. 1992 Jun;33(6):825-30.
189. Central mechanisms in pain. Urban MO1, Gebhart GF. Med Clin North Am. 1999 May;83(3):585-96.
190. Neuronal involvement in the intestinal effects of Clostridium difficile toxin A and Vibrio cholerae enterotoxin in rat ileum. Castagliuolo I *et al.*, . Gastroenterology. 1994 Sep;107(3):657-65.
191. Centers for Disease Control and Prevention http://www.cdc.gov/ncbddd/autism/data.html
192. Anxiety, sensory over-responsivity, and gastrointestinal problems in children with autism spectrum disorders. Mazurek MO, *et al.*, J Abnorm Child Psychol. 2013.
193. Aluminum and Glyphosate Can Synergistically Induce Pineal Gland Pathology: Connection to Gut Dysbiosis and Neurological Disease. Stephanie Seneff *et al.*, Agricultural Sciences. Vol.06 No.01(2015), Article ID:53106,28 pages 10.4236/as.2015.61005
194. Commensal bacteria (normal microflora), mucosal immunity and chronic inflammatory and autoimmune diseases. Tlaskalová-Hogenová H *et al.*, Immunol Lett. 2004 May 15;93(2-3):97-108.
195. Toward Effective Probiotics for Autism and Other Neurodevelopmental Disorders Jack A. Gilbert *et al.*, Cell, Volume 155, Issue 7, 19 December 2013, Pages 1446–1448

196. Reduced Incidence of Prevotella and Other Fermenters in Intestinal Microflora of Autistic Children. Dae-Wook Kang *et al.*, Plos one, July 3, 2013DOI: 10.1371/journal.pone.0068322. http://journals.plos.org/plosone/article?id=10.1371/journal.pone.0068322

197. How does peripheral lipopolysaccharide induce gene expression in the brain of rats? A.K Singh, , Y Jiang. Toxicology Volume 201, Issues 1–3, 1 September 2004, Pages 197–207

198. Mercury in first-cut baby hair of children with autism versus typically-developing children. JB Adams *et al.*, Toxicological & Environmental Chemistry. Volume 90, Issue 4, 2008; pages 739-753

199. The role of epigenetic change in autism spectrum disorders. Yuk Jing Loke *et al.*, Front. Neurol., 26 May 2015

200. Wong CCY, Meaburn EL, Ronald A, et al. Methylomic analysis of monozygotic twins discordant for autism spectrum disorder and related behavioural traits. Molecular Psychiatry. 2014;19(4):495-503. doi:10.1038/mp.2013.41.

201. Wong CCY, Meaburn EL, Ronald A, et al. Methylomic analysis of monozygotic twins discordant for autism spectrum disorder and related behavioural traits. Molecular Psychiatry. 2014;19(4):495-503. doi:10.1038/mp.2013.41.

202. Carding, Simon *et al.*, . "Dysbiosis of the gut microbiota in disease." Microbial Ecology in Health and Disease [Online], 26 (2015): n. pag. Web. 9 Mar. 2016

203. Romano-Keeler J, Weitkamp J-H. Maternal influences on fetal microbial colonization and immune development. Pediatric research. 2015;77(0):189-195. doi:10.1038/pr.2014.163.

204. A maternal gluten-free diet reduces inflammation and diabetes incidence in the offspring of NOD mice. Hansen CH *et al.*, Diabetes. 2014 Aug;63(8):2821-32. doi: 10.2337/db13-1612. Epub 2014 Apr 2.

205. Maternal separation disrupts the integrity of the intestinal microflora in infant rhesus monkeys. Bailey MT, Coe CL. Dev Psychobiol. 1999 Sep; 35(2):146-55.

206. De la Monte SM, Wands JR. Alzheimer's Disease Is Type 3 Diabetes–Evidence Reviewed. Journal of diabetes science and technology (Online). 2008;2(6):1101-1113.
207. Hill JM, Bhattacharjee S, Pogue AI, Lukiw WJ. The Gastrointestinal Tract Microbiome and Potential Link to Alzheimer's Disease. Frontiers in Neurology. 2014;5:43. doi:10.3389/fneur.2014.00043.
208. De la Monte SM, Wands JR. Alzheimer's Disease Is Type 3 Diabetes–Evidence Reviewed. Journal of diabetes science and technology (Online). 2008;2(6):1101-1113.
209. Hill JM, Bhattacharjee S, Pogue AI, Lukiw WJ. The Gastrointestinal Tract Microbiome and Potential Link to Alzheimer's Disease. Frontiers in Neurology. 2014;5:43. doi:10.3389/fneur.2014.00043.
210. Gut bacteria and brain function: The challenges of a growing field. Philip W. J. Burnet. PNAS vol. 109 no. 4 > Philip W. J. Burnet, E175, doi: 10.1073/pnas.1118654109

Chapter Eleven
211. Is eating behavior manipulated by the gastrointestinal microbiota? Evolutionary pressures and potential mechanisms. Joe Alcock *et al.*, BioEssays Volume 36, Issue 10, pages 940–949, October 2014
212. Is eating behavior manipulated by the gastrointestinal microbiota? Evolutionary pressures and potential mechanisms. Joe Alcock et al., BioEssays Volume 36, Issue 10, pages 940–949, October 2014
213. Intestinal permeability, gut-bacterial dysbiosis, and behavioral markers of alcohol-dependence severity. Sophie Leclercq *et al.*, PNAS. October 21, 2014 vol. 111 no. 42
214. Low-molecular-weight polyethylene glycol as a probe of gastrointestinal permeability after alcohol ingestion. Robinson GM *et al.*, Dig Dis Sci. 1981 Nov;26(11):971-7.
215. Kirpich, Irina A. et al. "Probiotics Restore Bowel Flora and Improve Liver Enzymes in Human Alcohol-Induced Liver Injury: A Pilot Study." Alcohol (Fayetteville, N.Y.) 42.8 (2008): 675–682. PMC. Web. 9 Mar. 2016.

216. Kirpich, Irina A. et al. "Probiotics Restore Bowel Flora and Improve Liver Enzymes in Human Alcohol-Induced Liver Injury: A Pilot Study." Alcohol (Fayetteville, N.Y.) 42.8 (2008): 675–682. PMC. Web. 9 Mar. 2016.

217. Modulation of human dendritic cell phenotype and function by probiotic bacteria. Hart AL *et al.*, Gut. 2004 Nov;53(11):1602-9.

218. Ghrelin system in alcohol-dependent subjects: role of plasma ghrelin levels in alcohol drinking and craving. Leggio L *et al.*, Addict Biol. 2012 Mar;17(2):452-64. doi: 10.1111/j.1369-1600.2010.00308.x. Epub 2011 Mar 11.

219. Do Gut Bacteria Rule Our Minds? In an Ecosystem Within Us, Microbes Evolved to Sway Food Choices. By Jeffrey Norris on August 15, 2014. USCF News Center.

220. A microbial symbiosis factor prevents intestinal inflammatory disease. Mazmanian SK, Round JL, Kasper DL. Nature. 2008 May 29;453(7195):620-5. doi: 10.1038/nature07008.

221. Influence of microbial species on small intestinal myoelectric activity and transit in germ-free rats. Einar Husebye, Per M. Hellström, Frank Sundler, Jie Chen, Tore Midtvedt. American Journal of Physiology - Gastrointestinal and Liver Physiology Published 1 March 2001 Vol. 280 no. 3, G368-G380 DOI:

222. Lactobacillus farciminis treatment suppresses stress induced visceral hypersensitivity: a possible action through interaction with epithelial cell cytoskelcton contraction. Ait-Belgnaoui A, Han W, Lamine F, Eutamene H, Fioramonti J, Bueno L, and Theodorou V. Gut. 2006 Aug; 55(8): 1090–1094.

Chapter Twelve
223. Zhang Y, Proenca R, Maffei M, Barone M, Leopold L, Friedman JM. Positional cloning of the mouse obese gene and its human homologue. Nature 1994; 372: 425–432.

224. Tiaka, Elisavet K. et al. "Unraveling the Link between Leptin, Ghrelin and Different Types of Colitis." Annals of Gastroenterology : Quarterly Publication of the Hellenic Society of Gastroenterology 24.1 (2011): 20–28. Print.
225. Reduction of T cell–derived ghrelin enhances proinflammatory cytokine expression: implications for age-associated increases in inflammation. Vishwa D. Dixit *et al.,* www.bloodjournal.org. May 21, 2009; Blood: 113 (21)
226. The intricate interface between immune and metabolic regulation: a role for leptin in the pathogenesis of multiple sclerosis? Giuseppe Matarese1, Claudio Procaccini and Veronica De Rosa. October 2008 Journal of Leukocyte Biology vol. 84 no. 4 893-899
227. Novel Connections Between the Neuroendocrine and Immune Systems: The Ghrelin Immunoregulatory Network. Dennis D. Taub. ScienceDirect. Vitamins & Hormones, Volume 77, 2007, Pages 325–346
228. The role of leptin and ghrelin in the regulation of food intake and body weight in humans: a review. M. D. Klok, S. Jakobsdottir andM. L. Drent. Obesity Reviews, Volume 8, Issue 1, pages 21–34, January 2007
229. Frost, Gary S. et al. "Impacts of Plant-Based Foods in Ancestral Hominin Diets on the Metabolism and Function of Gut Microbiota In Vitro." mBio 5.3 (2014): e00853–14. PMC. Web. 10 Mar. 2016.
230. New Revelations Support Diet and Exercise to Reverse Leptin Resistance, Thereby Promoting a Healthy Weight. Dr Mercola. Sourced 10 March 2016. http://articles.mercola.com/sites/articles/archive/2012/10/29/leptin-resistance.aspx

Chapter Thirteen

231. Personalized Nutrition by Prediction of Glycemic Responses. David Zeevi *et al.,* Cell, Volume 163, Issue 5, p1079–1094, 19 November 2015
232. Personalized Nutrition by Prediction of Glycemic Responses. David Zeevi et al., Cell, Volume 163, Issue 5, p1079–1094, 19 November 2015

233. ISOLATION AND CHARECTERIZATION OF PROBIOTIC BACTERIA FROM HUMAN MILK. Vaibhav Bhatt *et al.*, International journal of pharmaceutical science and health care 06/2012; 3(2):62-70.

234. Review article: probiotics and prebiotics in irritable bowel syndrome. Spiller R. Aliment Pharmacol Ther. 2008 Aug 15;28(4):385-96. doi: 10.1111/j.1365-2036.2008.03750.x. Epub 2008 Jun 4

235. Linking long-term dietary patterns with gut microbial enterotypes. Wu GD *et al.*, Science. 2011 Oct 7;334(6052):105-8. doi: 10.1126/science.1208344. Epub 2011 Sep 1.

236. Hemarajata P, Versalovic J. Effects of probiotics on gut microbiota: mechanisms of intestinal immunomodulation and neuromodulation. Therapeutic Advances in Gastroenterology. 2013;6(1):39-51. doi:10.1177/1756283X12459294.

237. Hemarajata P, Versalovic J. Effects of probiotics on gut microbiota: mechanisms of intestinal immunomodulation and neuromodulation. Therapeutic Advances in Gastroenterology. 2013;6(1):39-51. doi:10.1177/1756283X12459294.

238. The Four Best Probiotics For Hashimoto's. The Role of the Gut By Dr. Izabella Wentz, Pharm D. thyroidpharmacist.com

239. Brenta G. Why Can Insulin Resistance Be a Natural Consequence of Thyroid Dysfunction? Journal of Thyroid Research. 2011;2011:152850. doi:10.4061/2011/152850.

240. Kalra S, Unnikrishnan AG, Sahay R. The hypoglycemic side of hypothyroidism. Indian Journal of Endocrinology and Metabolism. 2014;18(1):1-3. doi:10.4103/2230-8210.126517.

241. Gut microbiome, gut function, and probiotics: Implications for health. Hajela N *et al.*, Indian J Gastroenterol. 2015 Mar;34(2):93-107. doi: 10.1007/s12664-015-0547-6. Epub 2015 Apr 29.

242. The development of probiotic treatment in obesity: a review. Review article Mekkes MC, et al. Benef Microbes. 2014 Mar;5(1):19-28. doi: 10.3920/BM2012.0069.

243. Kau AL, Ahern PP, Griffin NW, Goodman AL, Gordon JI. Human nutrition, the gut microbiome, and immune system: envisioning the future. Nature. 2011;474(7351):327-336. doi:10.1038/nature10213.

244. Lactobacillus brevis OK56 ameliorates high-fat diet-induced obesity in mice by inhibiting NF-κB activation and gut microbial LPS production. Kyung-Ah Kim et al., Journal of Functional Foods. Volume 13, March 2015, Pages 183–191

245. Frank, Daniel N. et al. "Molecular-Phylogenetic Characterization of Microbial Community Imbalances in Human Inflammatory Bowel Diseases." Proceedings of the National Academy of Sciences of the United States of America 104.34 (2007): 13780–13785. PMC. Web. 10 Mar. 2016.

246. Frank DN, St. Amand AL, Feldman RA, Boedeker EC, Harpaz N, Pace NR. Molecular-phylogenetic characterization of microbial community imbalances in human inflammatory bowel diseases. Proceedings of the National Academy of Sciences of the United States of America. 2007;104(34):13780-13785. doi:10.1073/pnas.0706625104.

247. A microbial symbiosis factor prevents intestinal inflammatory disease. Mazmanian SK, Round JL, Kasper DL. Nature. 2008 May 29;453(7195):620-5. doi: 10.1038/nature07008.

248. Clinical trial: the effects of a fermented milk product containing Bifidobacterium lactis DN-173 010 on abdominal distension and gastrointestinal transit in irritable bowel syndrome with constipation. Agrawal A et al., Aliment Pharmacol Ther. 2009 Jan;29(1):104-14. doi: 10.1111/j.1365-2036.2008.03853.x. Epub 2008 Sep 17.

249. Mueller C, Macpherson AJ. Layers of mutualism with commensal bacteria protect us from intestinal inflammation. Gut. 2006;55(2):276-284. doi:10.1136/gut.2004.054098.

250. Recognition of commensal microflora by toll-like receptors is required for intestinal homeostasis. Rakoff-Nahoum S et al., Cell. 2004 Jul 23;118(2):229-41.

251. Kirpich IA, Solovieva NV, Leikhter SN, et al. Probiotics Restore Bowel Flora and Improve Liver Enzymes in Human Alcohol-Induced Liver Injury: A Pilot Study. Alcohol (Fayetteville, NY). 2008;42(8):675-682. doi:10.1016/j.alcohol.2008.08.006.

252. Kirpich IA, Solovieva NV, Leikhter SN, et al. Probiotics Restore Bowel Flora and Improve Liver Enzymes in Human Alcohol-Induced Liver Injury: A Pilot Study. Alcohol (Fayetteville, NY). 2008;42(8):675-682. doi:10.1016/j.alcohol.2008.08.006.

253. Modulation of human dendritic cell phenotype and function by probiotic bacteria. Hart AL et al., Gut. 2004 Nov;53(11):1602-9.

254. Biedermann L, Zeitz J, Mwinyi J, et al. Smoking Cessation Induces Profound Changes in the Composition of the Intestinal Microbiota in Humans. Heimesaat MM, ed. PLoS ONE. 2013;8(3):e59260. doi:10.1371/journal.pone.0059260.

255. Kim H-J, Kim HY, Lee S-Y, Seo J-H, Lee E, Hong S-J. Clinical efficacy and mechanism of probiotics in allergic diseases. Korean Journal of Pediatrics. 2013;56(9):369-376. doi:10.3345/kjp.2013.56.9.369.

256. A systematic review and meta-analysis of probiotics for the treatment of allergic rhinitis. Zajac AE1, Adams AS1, Turner JH1. Int Forum Allergy Rhinol. 2015 Jun;5(6):524-32. doi: 10.1002/alr.21492. Epub 2015 Apr 20.

257. Synbiotics prevent asthma-like symptoms in infants with atopic dermatitis. van der Aa LB et al., Allergy. 2011 Feb;66(2):170-7. doi: 10.1111/j.1398-9995.2010.02416.x.

258. Peanut allergies: Australian study into probiotics offers hope for possible cure. By medical reporter Sophie Scott. Updated 29 Jan 2015, 3:29am. Sourced 10 March 2016. http://www.abc.net.au/

259. Wang J, Tang H, Zhang C, et al. Modulation of gut microbiota during probiotic-mediated attenuation of metabolic syndrome in high fat diet-fed mice. The ISME Journal. 2015;9(1):1-15. doi:10.1038/ismej.2014.99.

260. Lactobacillus acidophilus modulates intestinal pain and induces opioid and cannabinoid receptors. Rousseaux C et al., Nat Med. 2007 Jan;13(1):35-7. Epub 2006 Dec 10.

261. Bhattacharjee S, Lukiw WJ. Alzheimer's disease and the microbiome. Frontiers in Cellular Neuroscience. 2013;7:153. doi:10.3389/fncel.2013.00153.

262. Ingestion of Lactobacillus strain regulates emotional behavior and central GABA receptor expression in a mouse via the vagus nerve. Bravo JA, et al. Proc Natl Acad Sci U S A. 2011 Sep 20;108(38):16050-5. doi: 10.1073/pnas.1102999108. Epub 2011 Aug 29.

263. Gut bacteria and brain function: The challenges of a growing field. Philip W. J. Burnet. PNAS vol. 109 no. 4 > Philip W. J. Burnet, E175, doi: 10.1073/pnas.1118654109

264. Deregulation of excitatory neurotransmission underlying synapse failure in Alzheimer's disease. Paula-Lima AC et al., J Neurochem. 2013 Jul;126(2):191-202. doi: 10.1111/jnc.12304. Epub 2013 May 28.

265. A randomized, double-blind, placebo-controlled pilot study of a probiotic in emotional symptoms of chronic fatigue syndrome. Rao AV et al., Gut Pathog. 2009 Mar 19;1(1):6. doi: 10.1186/1757-4749-1-6.

266. Foster JA. Gut Feelings: Bacteria and the Brain. Cerebrum: the Dana Forum on Brain Science. 2013;2013:9.

267. That gut feeling. Dr. Siri Carpenter. September 2012, Vol 43, No. 8. Print version: page 50. American Psychological Association.

268. Microbiota modulate behavioral and physiological abnormalities associated with neurodevelopmental disorders. Hsiao EY et al., Cell. 2013 Dec 19;155(7):1451-63. doi: 10.1016/j.cell.2013.11.024. Epub 2013 Dec 5.

269. The intestinal barrier and its regulation by neuroimmune factors. Keita AV1, Söderholm JD. Neurogastroenterol Motil. 2010 Jul;22(7):718-33. doi: 10.1111/j.1365-2982.2010.01498.x. Epub 2010 Apr 9.

270. Bhattacharjee S, Lukiw WJ. Alzheimer's disease and the microbiome. Frontiers in Cellular Neuroscience. 2013;7:153. doi:10.3389/fncel.2013.00153.

271. Bhattacharjee S, Lukiw WJ. Alzheimer's disease and the microbiome. Frontiers in Cellular Neuroscience. 2013;7:153. doi:10.3389/fncel.2013.00153.

272. The role of microbes and autoimmunity in the pathogenesis of neuropsychiatric illness. Hornig M. Curr Opin Rheumatol. 2013 Jul;25(4):488-795. doi: 10.1097/BOR.0b013e32836208de.

273. Anxiogenic effect of subclinical bacterial infection in mice in the absence of overt immune activation. Lyte M1, Varcoe JJ, Bailey MT. Physiol Behav. 1998 Aug;65(1):63-8.

274. Innate Immune System and Inflammation in Alzheimer's Disease: From Pathogenesis to Treatment. Serpente M et al., Neuroimmunomodulation 2014;21:79-87 (DOI:10.1159/000356529)

275. Hill JM, Lukiw WJ. Microbial-generated amyloids and Alzheimer's disease (AD). Frontiers in Aging Neuroscience. 2015;7:9. doi:10.3389/fnagi.2015.00009.

276. Gut bacteria and brain function: The challenges of a growing field. Philip W. J. Burnet. PNAS vol. 109 no. 4 > Philip W. J. Burnet, E175, doi: 10.1073/pnas.1118654109

277. Fermented foods, neuroticism, and social anxiety: An interaction model. Matthew R. Hilimire, Jordan E. DeVylder, Catherine A. Forestell. Psychiatry Research August 15, 2015Volume 228, Issue 2, Pages 203–208

278. Fermented foods, neuroticism, and social anxiety: An interaction model. Matthew R. Hilimire, Jordan E. DeVylder, Catherine A. Forestell. Psychiatry Research August 15, 2015Volume 228, Issue 2, Pages 203–208

279. Probiotic Lactobacillus casei strain Shirota prevents indomethacin-induced small intestinal injury: involvement of lactic acid. Watanabe T et al., Am J Physiol Gastrointest Liver Physiol. 2009 Sep;297(3):G506-13. doi: 10.1152/ajpgi.90553.2008. Epub 2009 Jul 9.

280. Thomas CM, Hong T, van Pijkeren JP, et al. Histamine Derived from Probiotic Lactobacillus reuteri Suppresses TNF via Modulation of PKA and ERK Signaling. Heimesaat MM, ed. PLoS ONE. 2012;7(2):e31951. doi:10.1371/journal.pone.0031951.

281. Lactobacillus GG in the prevention of gastrointestinal and respiratory tract infections in children who attend day care centers: A randomized, double-blind, placebo-controlled trial. Iva Hojsak et al., Clinical Nutrition. June 2010Volume 29, Issue 3, Pages 312–316

282. Endothelial Nitric Oxide Synthase in Vascular Disease. From Marvel to Menace. American Heart Association. Sourced 10 March 2016.
http://m.circ.ahajournals.org/content/113/13/1708.full

283. Generation of NO by probiotic bacteria in the gastrointestinal tract. Sobko T et al., Free Radic Biol Med. 2006 Sep 15;41(6):985-91. Epub 2006 Jul 4.

284. Biagi E, Candela M, Fairweather-Tait S, Franceschi C, Brigidi P. Ageing of the human metaorganism: the microbial counterpart. Age. 2012;34(1):247-267. doi:10.1007/s11357-011-9217-5.

285. Microbiome therapy gains market traction. Sara Reardon. Nature, 13 May 2014

286. Ursell LK, Knight R. Xenobiotics and the human gut microbiome: metatranscriptomics reveal the active players. Cell metabolism. 2013;17(3):317-318. doi:10.1016/j.cmet.2013.02.013.

287. Exploring gut microbes in human health and disease: Pushing the envelope. Jun Suna, Eugene B. Chang. ScienceDirect. doi:10.1016/j.gendis.2014.08.001. Genes & Diseases. Volume 1, Issue 2, December 2014, Pages 132–139

288. Is it time for a metagenomic basis of therapeutics? Haiser HJ, Turnbaugh PJ. Science. 2012 Jun 8;336(6086):1253-5. doi: 10.1126/science.1224396. Epub 2012 Jun 6.

289. 288. Systems Modeling of Interactions between Mucosal Immunity and the Gut Microbiome during Clostridium difficile Infection. Andrew Leber,Monica Viladomiu, Raquel Hontecillas,Vida Abedi, Casandra Philipson, Stefan Hoops, Brad Howard, and Josep Bassaganya-Riera1. PLoS One. 2015; 10(7): e0134849. Published online 2015 Jul 31. doi: 10.1371/journal.pone.0134849

290. Rohlke F, Stollman N. Fecal microbiota transplantation in relapsing Clostridium difficile infection. Therapeutic Advances in Gastroenterology. 2012;5(6):403-420. doi:10.1177/1756283X12453637.
291. http://www.openbiome.org/
292. Hill JM, Bhattacharjee S, Pogue AI, Lukiw WJ. The Gastrointestinal Tract Microbiome and Potential Link to Alzheimer's Disease. Frontiers in Neurology. 2014;5:43. doi:10.3389/fneur.2014.00043.
293. Fermented foods, neuroticism, and social anxiety: An interaction model. Matthew R. Hilimire, Jordan E. DeVylder, Catherine A. Forestell. Psychiatry Research August 15, 2015Volume 228, Issue 2, Pages 203–208
294. Abdallah Ismail N, Ragab SH, Abd ElBaky A, Shoeib ARS, Alhosary Y, Fekry D. Frequency of Firmicutes and Bacteroidetes in gut microbiota in obese and normal weight Egyptian children and adults. Archives of Medical Science : AMS. 2011;7(3):501-507. doi:10.5114/aoms.2011.23418.
295. http://nutritionfacts.org/video/tipping-the-balance-of-firmicutes-to-bacteroidetes/
296. Conlon MA, Bird AR. The Impact of Diet and Lifestyle on Gut Microbiota and Human Health. Nutrients. 2015;7(1):17-44. doi:10.3390/nu7010017.
297. Up-regulating the human intestinal microbiome using whole plant foods, polyphenols, and/or fiber. Tuohy KM et al., J Agric Food Chem. 2012 Sep 12;60(36):8776-82. doi: 10.1021/jf2053959. Epub 2012 Jun 12.
298. Personalized Nutrition by Prediction of Glycemic Responses. David Zeevi et al., Cell, Volume 163, Issue 5, p1079–1094, 19 November 2015
299. Personalized Nutrition by Prediction of Glycemic Responses. David Zeevi et al., Cell, Volume 163, Issue 5, p1079–1094, 19 November 2015
300. Artificial sweeteners induce glucose intolerance by altering the gut microbiota. Jotham suez et al., Nature aop, (2014) | doi:10.1038/nature13793

301. Dietary emulsifiers impact the mouse gut microbiota promoting colitis and metabolic syndrome. Benoit Chassaing et al., Nature 519, 92–96 (05 March 2015) doi:10.1038/nature14232. Published online 25 February 2015. Sourced 10 March 2016.
302. Food preservatives linked to obesity and gut disease. Sara Reardon. Nature, 25 February 2015
303. Possible neurologic effects of aspartame, a widely used food additive. T J Maher and R J Wurtman. Environ Health Perspect. 1987 Nov; 75: 53–57. PMCID: PMC1474447. Research Article
304. Is There Toxic Waste In Your Body? by Mark Hyman, MD. http://drhyman.com/blog/2010/05/19/is-there-toxic-waste-in-your-body-2/. Sourced 11 March 2016
305. The prevention and control the type-2 diabetes by changing lifestyle and dietary pattern. Mohammad Asif. J Educ Health Promot. 2014; 3: 1. Published online 2014 Feb 21. doi: 10.4103/2277-9531.127541
306. The Association of Maternal Obesity and Diabetes With Autism and Other Developmental Disabilities. Mengying Li et al., Paediatrics, February 2016.
307. Nutrient Power: Heal Your Biochemistry and Heal Your Brain. William J. Walsh. Skyhorse Publishing; updated edition (6 May 2014).
308. Artificial sweeteners induce glucose intolerance by altering the gut microbiota. Jotham suez et al., Nature aop, (2014) | doi:10.1038/nature13793
309. Dietary emulsifiers impact the mouse gut microbiota promoting colitis and metabolic syndrome. Benoit Chassaing et al., Nature 519, 92–96 (05 March 2015) doi:10.1038/nature14232. Published online 25 February 2015. Sourced 10 March 2016.
310. Food preservatives linked to obesity and gut disease. Sara Reardon. Nature, 25 February 2015

311. The Prevalence of Antibodies against Wheat and Milk Proteins in Blood Donors and Their Contribution to Neuroimmune Reactivities. Aristo Vojdani et al., Nutrients. 2014 Jan; 6(1): 15–36. Published online 2013 Dec 19. doi: 10.3390/nu6010015

312. Milk proteins and human health: A1/A2 milk hypothesis. Monika Sodhi et al., Indian J Endocrinol Metab. 2012 Sep-Oct; 16(5): 856. doi: 10.4103/2230-8210.100685

313. Cade, Robert , Privette, Malcolm , Fregly, Melvin , Rowland, Neil , Sun, Zhongjie , Zele, Virginia, Wagemaker, Herbert and Edelstein, Charlotte(2000) 'Autism and Schizophrenia: Intestinal Disorders', Nutritional Neuroscience, 3: 1, 57 — 72

314. Milk--the promoter of chronic Western diseases. Melnik BC. Med Hypotheses. 2009 Jun;72(6):631-9. doi: 10.1016/j.mehy.2009.01.008. Epub 2009 Feb 15.

315. Ischaemic heart disease, Type 1 diabetes, and cow milk A1 beta-casein. Laugesen M1, Elliott R. N Z Med J. 2003 Jan 24;116(1168):U295.

316. Mucosal reactivity to cow's milk protein in coeliac disease. G Kristjánsson et al., Clin Exp Immunol. 2007 Mar; 147(3): 449–455. doi: 10.1111/j.1365-2249.2007.03298.x

317. Gluten and wheat intolerance today: are modern wheat strains involved? de Lorgeril M, Salen P. Int J Food Sci Nutr. 2014 Aug;65(5):577-81. doi: 10.3109/09637486.2014.886185. Epub 2014 Feb 13.

318. http://thyroidpharmacist.com/

319. Differentiation between Celiac Disease, Nonceliac Gluten Sensitivity, and Their Overlapping with Crohn's Disease: A Case Series. Aristo Vojdani 1 , 2 ,and David Perlmutter 3. Case Reports Immunol. 2013; 2013: 248482.

320. Published online 2013 Jan 27. doi: 10.1155/2013/248482

321. Gluten sensitivity in multiple sclerosis: experimental myth or clinical truth? Shor DB et al., Ann N Y Acad Sci. 2009 Sep;1173:343-9. doi: 10.1111/j.1749-6632.2009.04620.x.

322. Cross-Reaction between Gliadin and Different Food and Tissue AntigensAristo Vojdani1,2, Igal Tarash1. Food and Nutrition Sciences. Vol.4 No.1(2013), Paper ID 26626, 13 pages DOI:10.4236/fns.2013.41005

323. Cross-Reaction between Gliadin and Different Food and Tissue AntigensAristo Vojdani1,2, Igal Tarash1. Food and Nutrition Sciences. Vol.4 No.1(2013), Paper ID 26626, 13 pages DOI:10.4236/fns.2013.41005

324. The effect of glyphosate on potential pathogens and beneficial members of poultry microbiota in vitro. Shehata AA et al., Curr Microbiol. 2013 Apr;66(4):350-8. doi: 10.1007/s00284-012-0277-2. Epub 2012 Dec 9.

325. Aluminum and Glyphosate Can Synergistically Induce Pineal Gland Pathology: Connection to Gut Dysbiosis and Neurological Disease. Stephanie Seneff, Nancy Swanson, Chen Li. Agricultural Sciences. Vol.6 No.1(2015), Paper ID 53106, 29 pages. DOI:10.4236/as.2015.61005

326. Republished study: long-term toxicity of a Roundup herbicide and a Roundup-tolerant genetically modified maize. Gilles-Eric Séralini et al., Environmental Sciences EuropeBridging Science and Regulation at the Regional and European Level201426:14. DOI: 10.1186/s12302-014-0014-5© Séralini et al.; licensee Springer 2014 Received: 22 March 2014Accepted: 16 May 2014Published: 24 June 2014

327. Low-molecular-weight polyethylene glycol as a probe of gastrointestinal permeability after alcohol ingestion. Robinson GM et al., Dig Dis Sci. 1981 Nov;26(11):971-7.

328. Food, mood and health: a neurobiologic outlook. C. Prasad. Braz J Med Biol Res, December 1998, Volume 31(12) 1517-1527

329. Ingestion of Lactobacillus strain regulates emotional behavior and central GABA receptor expression in a mouse via the vagus nerve. Javier A. Bravo, PNAS, vol. 108 no. 38 > Javier A. Bravo, 16050–16055

330. Long-term vitamin D3 supplementation is more effective than vitamin D2 in maintaining serum 25-hydroxyvitamin D status over the winter months. Logan VF et al., Br J Nutr. 2013 Mar 28;109(6):1082-8. doi: 10.1017/S0007114512002851. Epub 2012 Jul 11.

331. The role of the posterior cingulate cortex in cognition and disease. Robert Leech and David J. Sharp. Brain. 2014 Jan; 137(1): 12–32. Published online 2013 Jul 18. doi: 10.1093/brain/awt162

332. Mindfulness: An Emerging Treatment for Smoking and other Addictions? Judson Brewer and Lori Pbert. Journal of Family Medicine. Received: August 26, 2015; Accepted: September 02, 2015; Published: September 03, 2015

333. Self-Regulation and Depletion of Limited Resources: Does Self-Control Resemble a Muscle? Mark Muraven and Roy F. Baumeister. Psychological Bulletin Copyright 2000 by the American Psychological Association, Inc. 2000, Vol. 126, No. 2, 247-259

334. Mindfulness: An Emerging Treatment for Smoking and other Addictions? Judson Brewer and Lori Pbert. Journal of Family Medicine. Received: August 26, 2015; Accepted: September 02, 2015; Published: September 03, 2015

335. Meditation leads to reduced default mode network activity beyond an active task. Kathleen A. Garrison. Cognitive, Affective, & Behavioral Neuroscience September 2015, Volume 15, Issue 3, pp 712-720

336. A randomized controlled trial of smartphone-based mindfulness training for smoking cessation: a study protocol. Kathleen A Garrison et al., BMC Psychiatry201515:83 DOI: 10.1186/s12888-015-0468-z© Garrison et al.; licensee BioMed Central. 2015. Received: 13 January 2015Accepted: 8 April 2015Published: 14 April 2015

337. http://www.ted.com/speakers/judson_brewer

Chapter Fourteen
338. Anti-fungal effect of berberine on Candida albicans by microcalorimetry with correspondence analysis. Yanling Zhao et al., Journal of Thermal Analysis and Calorimetry October 2010, Volume 102, Issue 1, pp 49-55

339. [Changes of metabolic indices caused by berberin and extract, obtained from the bark of Phellodendron lavalei, introduced in subtropic regions of Georgia, in streptozotocin induced diabetic rats. Article in Russian]. Meskheli MB et al., published in English Georgian Med News. 2011 Feb;(191):61-8.

340. An examination of antibacterial and antifungal properties of constituents described in traditional Ulster cures and remedies. Simon Woods-Panzaru et al., Ulster Med J. 2009 Jan; 78(1): 13–15.

341. An examination of antibacterial and antifungal properties of constituents described in traditional Ulster cures and remedies. Simon Woods-Panzaru et al., Ulster Med J. 2009 Jan; 78(1): 13–15.

342. Investigating Antibacterial Effects of Garlic (Allium sativum) Concentrate and Garlic-Derived Organosulfur Compounds on Campylobacter jejuni by Using Fourier Transform Infrared Spectroscopy, Raman Spectroscopy, and Electron Microscopy. Xiaonan Lu et al., Appl Environ Microbiol. 2011 Aug; 77(15): 5257–5269. doi: 10.1128/AEM.02845-10

343. Garlic Proven 100 Times More Effective Than Antibiotics, Working In A Fraction of The Time. April McCarthy PreventDisease.com May 2, 2012. Sourced 11 March 2016

344. Herbal Therapy Is Equivalent to Rifaximin for the Treatment of Small Intestinal Bacterial Overgrowth. Victor Chedid, MD et al., Global Adv Health Med. 2014; 3(3): 16 -24

345. Inhibitory Actions of Glycyrrhizic Acid on Arylamine N-Acetyltransferase Activity in Strains of Helicobacter Pylori from Peptic Ulcer Patients. Jing G. Chung. Drug and Chemical Toxicology. Volume 21, Issue 3, 1998, pages 355-370

346. The treatment of atopic dermatitis with licorice gel. Saeedi M et al., J Dermatolog Treat. 2003 Sep;14(3):153-7.

347. Self-help interventions for depressive disorders and depressive symptoms: a systematic review. Amy J Morgan and Anthony F Jorm. Annals of General Psychiatry20087:13 DOI: 10.1186/1744-859X-7-13© Morgan and Jorm; licensee BioMed Central Ltd. 2008. Received: 08 April 2008Accepted: 19 August 2008Published: 19 August 2008

348. Find a Vitamin or Supplement. ST. JOHN'S WORT. http://www.webmd.com/

349. The bovine protein α-lactalbumin increases the plasma ratio of tryptophan to the other large neutral amino acids, and in vulnerable subjects raises brain serotonin activity, reduces cortisol concentration, and improves mood under stress. C Rob Markus et al., Am J Clin Nutr June 2000 vol. 71 no. 6 1536-1544

350. Ginger Extract (Zingiber Officinale) has Anti-Cancer and Anti-Inflammatory Effects on Ethionine-Induced Hepatoma Rats. Shafina Hanim Mohd Habib et al., Clinics. 2008 Dec; 63(6): 807–813. doi: 10.1590/S1807-59322008000600017

351. Traditional Indian spices and their health significance. Kamala Krishnaswamy MD. Asia Pac J Clin Nutr 2008;17(S1):265-268

352. Traditional Indian spices and their health significance. Kamala Krishnaswamy MD. Asia Pac J Clin Nutr 2008;17(S1):265-268

353. Potential Therapeutic Effects of Curcumin, the Anti-inflammatory Agent, Against Neurodegenerative, Cardiovascular, Pulmonary, Metabolic, Autoimmune and Neoplastic Diseases. Bharat B. Aggarwall and Kuzhuvelil B. Harikumar. Int J Biochem Cell Biol. Author manuscript; available in PMC 2010 Jan 1. Int J Biochem Cell Biol. 2009; 41(1): 40–59.Published online 2008 Jul 9. doi: 10.1016/j.biocel.2008.06.010.

354. Effect of NCB-02, atorvastatin and placebo on endothelial function, oxidative stress and inflammatory markers in patients with type 2 diabetes mellitus: a randomized, parallel-group, placebo-controlled, 8-week study. Usharani P et al., Drugs R D. 2008;9(4):243-50.

355. http://www.drugs.com/dexamethasone.html

356. Evaluation of antidepressant like activity of curcumin and its combination with fluoxetine and imipramine: an acute and chronic study. Sanmukhani J et al., Acta Pol Pharm. 2011 Sep-Oct;68(5):769-75.

357. Effect of curcumin on platelet aggregation and vascular prostacyclin synthesis. Srivastava R et al., Arzneimittelforschung. 1986 Apr;36(4):715-7.

358. Comparison of oxaliplatin- and curcumin-mediated antiproliferative effects in colorectal cell lines. Howells LM, Mitra A, Manson MM. Int J Cancer. 2007 Jul 1;121(1):175-83.

359. Effects of curcumin or dexamethasone on lung ischaemia–reperfusion injury in rats. J. Sun, European Respiratory Journal, March 1 2016 (Vol 47 Issue 3). http://crj.ersjournals.com/

360. Recent Developments in Delivery, Bioavailability, Absorption and Metabolism of Curcumin: the Golden Pigment from Golden Spice. Sahdeo Prasad, PhD et al., Cancer Res Treat. 2014 Jan; 46(1): 2–18. Published online 2014 Jan 15. doi: 10.4143/crt.2014.46.1.2

361. Bioavailability of curcumin: problems and promises. Anand P et al., Mol Pharm. 2007 Nov-Dec;4(6):807-18. Epub 2007 Nov 14.

362. Influence of piperine on the pharmacokinetics of curcumin in animals and human volunteers. Shoba G et al., Planta Med. 1998 May;64(4):353-6.

363. Anti-inflammatory activity of extracts from fruits, herbs and spices. Monika Mueller et al., Food Chemistry 122 (2010) 987–996. Contents lists available at ScienceDirectFood Chemistryjournal homepage: www.elsevier.com/locate/foodchem

364. Supplementation of Vitamin C Reduces Blood Glucose and Improves Glycosylated Hemoglobin in Type 2 Diabetes Mellitus: A Randomized, Double-Blind Study. Ganesh N. Dakhale et al., Adv Pharmacol Sci. 2011; 2011: 195271. Published online 2011 Dec 28. doi: 10.1155/2011/195271

365. Vitamin B12-Containing Plant Food Sources for Vegetarians. Fumio Watanabe et al., Nutrients. 2014 May; 6(5): 1861–1873.

366. Published online 2014 May 5. doi: 10.3390/nu6051861

367. Vitamin D regulation of immune function. Bikle DD. Vitam Horm. 2011;86:1-21. doi: 10.1016/B978-0-12-386960-9.00001-0.
368. Long-term vitamin D3 supplementation is more effective than vitamin D2 in maintaining serum 25-hydroxyvitamin D status over the winter months. Logan VF et al., Br J Nutr. 2013 Mar 28;109(6):1082-8. doi: 10.1017/S0007114512002851. Epub 2012 Jul 11.

Chapter Fifteen
369. Is olive oil really good for me? http://www.bbc.co.uk/programmes/articles/tWtLcz30LZm3Y Tk5VfZ307/is-olive-oil-really-good-for-me. Sourced 11 March 2016
370. The Link Between Nightshades, Chronic Pain and Inflammation. Elisha McFarland. Greenmedinfo. Com. Sunday, April 21st 2013 at 5:00 am. Sourced 11 march 2016
371. Is olive oil really good for me? http://www.bbc.co.uk/programmes/articles/tWtLcz30LZm3Y Tk5VfZ307/is-olive-oil-really-good-for-me. Sourced 11 March 2016
372. Impacts of Plant-Based Foods in Ancestral Hominin Diets on the Metabolism and Function of Gut Microbiota In Vitro. Gary S. Frost et al., mBio. 2014 May-Jun; 5(3): e00853-14. Published online 2014 May 20. doi: 10.1128/mBio.00853-14

Chapter Sixteen

373. Why do we have blood types? Carl Zimmer. 15 July 2014. http://www.bbc.com/future/story/20140715-why-do-we-have-blood-types. Sourced 11 march 2016

374. Association between the ABO blood group and the human intestinal microbiota composition. Harri Mäkivuokko et al., BMC Microbiol. 2012; 12: 94. Published online 2012 Jun 6. doi: 10.1186/1471-2180-12-94

Chapter Seventeen

375. The Effects of Diet on Inflammation: Emphasis on the Metabolic Syndrome. Dario Giugliano, MD, PhD et al., Journal of the American College of Cardiology. Volume 48, Issue 4, 15 August 2006, Pages 677–685.

376. Why Cancer and Inflammation? Seth Rakoff-Nahoum. Yale J Biol Med. 2006 Dec; 79(3-4): 123–130. Published online 2007 Oct.

377. Fruit Polyphenols and Their Effects on Neuronal Signaling and Behavior in Senescence. James A Joseph et al., ANNALS OF THE NEW YORK ACADEMY OF SCIENCES 1100(1):470-85 · MAY 2007.

378. Why Cancer and Inflammation? Seth Rakoff-Nahoum. Yale J Biol Med. 2006 Dec; 79(3-4): 123–130. Published online 2007 Oct.

379. Smoldering and polarized inflammation in the initiation and promotion of malignant disease. Frances Balkwill et al. http://web.mit.edu/jlee08/Public/Cancer/Lecture7/balkwill_REV_2005.pdf

380. Fruit Polyphenols and Their Effects on Neuronal Signaling and Behavior in Senescence. James A Joseph et al., ANNALS OF THE NEW YORK ACADEMY OF SCIENCES 1100(1):470-85 · MAY 2007.

381. Anti-inflammatory activity of extracts from fruits, herbs and spices. Monika Mueller et al., Food Chemistry 122 (2010) 987–996 Contents lists available atScienceDirectFood Chemistryjournal homepage: www.elsevier.com/locate/foodchem.

382. NEUROENDOCRINE REGULATION OF IMMUNITY
Jeanette I. Webster et al.,Annual Review of Immunology.
Vol. 20: 125-163 (Volume publication date April 2002).
DOI: 10.1146/annurev.immunol.20.082401.104914

Chapter Eighteen
383. Epithelial tight junctions in intestinal inflammation. Review
article Schulzke JD, et al. Ann N Y Acad Sci. 2009.
May;1165:294-300. doi: 10.1111/j.1749-6632.2009.04062.x.
384. Zonulin and Its Regulation of Intestinal Barrier Function:
The Biological Door to Inflammation, Autoimmunity, and
Cancer. Alessio Fasano. Physiological Reviews Published 1
January 2011 Vol. 91 no. 1, 151-175 DOI:
10.1152/physrev.00003.2008
385. Personalized Nutrition by Prediction of Glycemic Responses.
David Zeevi et al., Cell, Volume 163, Issue 5, p1079–1094,
19 November 2015
386. Vitamin B12-Containing Plant Food Sources for Vegetarians.
Fumio Watanabe et al., Nutrients. 2014 May; 6(5): 1861–
1873. Published online 2014 May 5. doi:
10.3390/nu6051861

#0111 - 160117 - C0 - 210/148/17 - PB - DID1721509